THE A B C OF PSYCHOLOGY

C K OGDEN

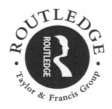

First published in 1929 by
Kegan Paul, Trench, Trubner & Co., Ltd.

Reprinted in 1999, 2001 by
Routledge

2 Park Square, Milton Park, Abingdon, Oxfordshire OX14 4RN
711 Third Avenue, New York, NY 10017

Transferred to Digital Printing 2006

First issued in paperback 2014

Routledge is an imprint of the Taylor and Francis Group, an informa company

British Library Cataloguing in Publication Data
A CIP catalogue record for this book
is available from the British Library

The A B C of Psychology
ISBN 13: 978-0-415-21036-2 (hbk)
ISBN 13: 978-0-415-75801-7 (pbk)

General Psychology: 38 Volumes
ISBN 978-0-415-21129-1
The International Library of Psychology: 204 Volumes
ISBN 978-0-415-19132-6

CONTENTS

PREFACE

A FEW years ago the word Psychology was a technicality covering a field of inquiry in which none but specialists and perhaps a few enterprising teachers were expected to take an interest. But at the present time it would be hard to find a general reader of current literature who has not at any rate browsed through one or more of the books on psychological topics which appear every other day.

There are, however, among these readers many who feel a difficulty in comparing and combining together the views, opinions, and information thus casually obtained. Although interested, they have no leisure for the study of voluminous works on first principles. They would like to read Shand's *Foundations of Character*, Marshall's *Consciousness*, Mitchell's *Structure and Growth of the Mind*, Wundt, Lipps, and Stumpf, Hobhouse's *Mind in Evolution*, Dumas' *Traité*, the *Analytic Psychology* of Professor Stout (having dipped perhaps into a volume with almost the same title by Dr Jung), Urban's exhaustive treatise on *Valuation*, Baldwin's *Thought and Things*, or the late Professor Ward's *Psychological Principles* ; but they have no ready means of discovering which is about what.

It seems probable, therefore, that many who are seriously approaching Psychology for the first time, and who are vaguely aware that many hundreds of important volumes have appeared since the last of these works was written, will welcome a brief account of the nucleus of accredited opinion from which the growing science is tending to develop. In what follows will be found an endeavour to deal with the subject in the simplest possible language, in the light of the most recent advances ; and to deal with it more concisely than has been done by any comprehensive introduction hitherto.

My object, however, has not merely been to cover the field on accepted lines. No conscientious teacher could to-day put his own Outline forward without taking account of the existence of admirable summaries such as those of Woodworth, McDougall, Pillsbury, and Yerkes. Each of these has its own advantages, and it would be no service to the public to attempt to combine their distinctive merits, or to forget that the two volumes of William James' *Principles* are generally accessible for reference with their abundance of unsurpassable descriptions. Nor can the physiological side of sense-perception, or the statistical handling of intelligence tests, for example, be usefully described in brief compass. For these the reader will be better advised to go direct to the original authorities, and I have therefore appended a short Bibliography of works available in the English language for his guidance in fuller reading.

It would be gratuitous to pretend that psychologists as a body are agreed on many fundamental issues. On this point the pages of *Psyche* or *The Psychological Review*, or the first hundred volumes of " The International Library of Psychology, Philosophy, and Scientific Method ", on which much of the present work is necessarily based, are alone conclusive. The reader who compares this Outline with right- and left-wing works such as Fox's *Educational Psychology* (1926) on the one hand, and Watson's *Behaviorism* (1925) on the other, will also be able to judge to what degree departure from tradition or undue conservatism is in evidence in the following pages.

There remains always the probability that some apparent differences of opinion are actually but differences in formulation ; this aspect of the problem, however, has already been discussed in *The Meaning of Meaning* (3rd Edition, 1930), to which the present work might serve as a stepping-stone for the linguistically inquisitive. On this occasion I have had the advantage of discussing numerous points with my former collaborator, Dr I. A. Richards of Magdalene College, to whose *Principles of Literary Criticism* I also owe much.

C. K. OGDEN.

MAGDALENE COLLEGE,
    CAMBRIDGE.

June, 1934.

THE ABC OF PSYCHOLOGY

CHAPTER I

PRELIMINARY

Reasons for the Study of Psychology.
There are four and a half good reasons for
studying Psychology seriously.

There are many more reasons for studying
it in other ways. It may help us to pose
more readily as profound thinkers, to write
more telling advertisements—or resist being
taken in by them—to detect failings in our
friends, and to discover new Wonders in
our Offspring. But none of these things will
carry the student through two hundred and
fifty pages. Fortunately there are stronger
motives.

1. WHAT ARE WE? Psychology is the only
means by which this momentous question
can ever be fully answered. Conchology
cannot do it, nor yet Ontology : nor Physics.
Physiology can only help us in part. Only by
a study of that portion of us which we call the

mind can we ever learn what the mind is. This may seem a simple saying, but its significance has only lately been generally accepted. Psychology is the youngest of the sciences, and the most attractive :

> " O latest born and loveliest vision far
> Of all Olympus' faded hierarchy "

says Keats in his " Ode to Psyche ". The study of the psyche, of mental processes, besides its universal appeal, has this further advantage that we each carry perpetually about with us all the subject matter which it requires.

2. WE GO WRONG. Even if we do not, we are always in a position to say with Richard Baxter : " there, but for the Grace of God, goes Richard ". And psychology is beginning to point out both how we may avoid disaster and how regain the right track. The labours of Gall, Esquirol, Carpenter, Maudsley, Charcot, Ribot, Hughlings Jackson, Stanley Hall, Goltz, Creighton, Ferrier, Havelock Ellis, Janet, Freud, Adler, Rivers, and a thousand others have already made modern psychotherapy a powerful resource against the worst afflictions to which man is liable.

3. WE CAN BE IMPROVED. If the reader was ever a child he will fully realize how much

room for improvement not only we, but our outworn educational methods, allow. " It is quite true," wrote Professor James Harvey Robinson in 1921, " that what we need is education, but something so different from what now passes as such that it needs a new name." And in the last twelve years the Walls of the World, the bounds of human imagination and knowledge, have again been swept back by the further triumphs of Einstein, Eddington, Compton, Rutherford, and Dirac ; while at the very heart of our being new and intricate mechanisms and possibilities are being revealed by fresh applications of such researches as those of Pavlov, Bose, Rowe, Cannon, Jaensch, Lashley, and the newer psycho-analysts. At the same time international, economic, and social affairs, and the contacts between minds, between types, races, and classes, which they entail, grow ever more bewildering. When confronted by these problems, or by our ignorance with regard to them, we must confess our inadequacy. We must learn how to learn —and our name is Legion. Democracy must face its problems. New millions of participants in the control of general affairs must now attempt to form personal opinions upon matters which were once left to a few. At the same time the complexity of these matters has immensely increased. The old view that the only access to a subject is through prolonged study of it, if true, has consequences for the immediate future which have not yet been faced. The alternative is to raise the level of communication through a direct study of its conditions, its dangers, and its difficulties. The practical side of this undertaking is, if communication be taken in its wide sense, education.

4. THE MIND IS A STARTING-POINT. Psychology ultimately provides a basis for all other studies—Ethics, Economics, Æsthetics, Ethnology, Grammar, Politics, and Mathematics. Even Physics is ultimately driven back on hypotheses which are essentially matters of psychological criticism and construction. All our research is the exercise of our thinking powers, and in the long run the test for thinking lies with those whose business it is to study the processes of thought. This has, of course, always been realized by those physicists whom the world acclaims as at once the most prudent and the most daring.

To turn to the science which seems the

most removed from Physics—namely Ethics.
As fashions have changed in psychology men's
theories of the good have followed them.
This is inevitable, for ever since the days of
Aristotle it has been agreed that only
experiences can be ' good ' or ' bad '. At
this point, however, it is worth warning the
reader who is approaching psychology for
the first time that he must not be disturbed
by the special associations which certain
simple terms such as *experience* (=' a terrible
experience '), *sensation* (cf. ' sensational '),
and even *perception* and *adaptation*, have
acquired in daily life and in the press. He
will soon get accustomed to their more
'general uses. Experiences, then, are what
we are ultimately assessing when we assign
ethical values, and in describing the differences between good and bad experiences
it is desirable to know how experiences may
differ. The most commonplace view—" The
greatest *happiness* of the greatest number "
—no less than the most transcendental,
" *Self*-realization ", depends upon discussions
which figure largely in every psychological
treatise.

Nor is the science of the Beautiful
(Æsthetics) capable of being divorced from

Psychology. What we are really talking about when we criticize a poem, a picture, or even a statue are essentially the states of mind (including pleasure, emotion, ecstasy, synæsthesis, and so forth) which they cause in us, so that the central problem of Æsthetics is to decide which of the states of mind that arise as our response to a given work of art are relevant.

Finally, as Mr Belloc wrote:

> " The Path of Life, men said, is hard and rough
> Only because we do not know enough.
> When Science has discovered something more
> We shall be happier than we were before."

If this be really true, Psychology, in virtue of its unique position among the sciences, would gain another half point.

The Subject Matter of Psychology. Clearly, however, Psychologizing is not one of the ' instincts '. It cannot be embarked on *ab ovo*, or from the cradle. Introspection (Lat. *introspicio*=look inward) is its main instrument, and a certain amount of training is necessary in introspection as in most other pursuits. Before commencing a detailed study we may make a brief preliminary survey of the field. The subject matter of Psychology is perhaps best indicated by an example.

As the reader reads these words he will probably agree that many things happen " in his mind ".

He *attends* to the marks on the paper, he *thinks* and *understands*, he takes up an *attitude*, he *remembers*, he is *interested* or *bored* as a consequence, his *instinct* of curiosity is perhaps aroused, or possibly he is *irritated* by the obscurity of the style. He *endeavours* to persevere, until eventually he feels *tired*, and to avoid pain he falls *asleep*. But even then he may *dream*, and on awakening may *forget* his dream—though if hypnotized he may rescue it from the *unconscious*.

All these are psychological events described in current psychological language, and in psychology we are either engaged in classifying such events and elaborating our descriptions of what takes place, or in seeking for their causes, *i.e.*, explaining why just that particular process took place at just that time in just that way.

The first of these, classification, is academic psychology—useful when wanted, but receding in favour of genetic (*Gk. genesis*=origin) and causal treatment. By genetic treatment is meant the treatment which seeks for light upon the things with which it deals

B

through the study of their origin, their
history, and their development.   When we
thus approach the mind we find that the importance of past history is far greater than
it is with physical processes.   In fact we
never think or feel or act quite freshly and
spontaneously, for the character of our thinking, our feeling, and our acting is always
due, in part at least, to the ways in which
we have thought and felt and acted in the
past.   What exactly this dependence in any
particular case may be is the main question
which psychology attempts to answer, and
it is chiefly in order to trace these connections
more easily that it adopts a special vocabulary.

Technical Distinctions.   Popular language in all matters that are connected with
the mind is apt to be vague and misleading.
Psychologists have   therefore   felt obliged
to introduce terms freer from irrelevant
associations than those in ordinary use, and
these often make the subject seem dry and
abstract to the beginner.   But if it is realized
that they are only names for what must
from the nature of the case be processes
familiar to everyone as part of ordinary
experience, a little patience is all that is
necessary for the mastery of current opinions.

Thus we find *Psychosis* ('state of mind', and sometimes 'abnormal state of mind': much as *phenomenon*='appearance', and sometimes 'abnormal appearance'), *Conation* (striving), *Volition* (will), *Affect* (feeling), *Cognition* (knowing), *Engram* (impression), *Presentation* (sensation), *Ideation* (thinking), *Hedonic tone* (pleasure-pain), *Endo-somatic* (inside the skin), *Cenesthesia* (sensibility of the whole body); and so on. Some of these terms will of course be found in the present work; others are not of much use.

Adaptation. From the most general standpoint, the business of the mind is to adapt the organism to its environment. The process of continual change from adaptation to adaptation is what is known as *Conation* (Lat. *conor*=try). In cases where there is conscious effort this process is popularly known as 'willing'. It is, however, now widely held that there is no essential difference, beyond a difference in complexity, between automatic responses to the environment and those responses which, owing to a conflict of tendencies, seem to involve the efforts of something which may be called the 'Will'. There are difficulties in admitting such an agent as the Will into psychology as a science, but on the view that all mental change is conative, we must of course admit that we are ' willing ' even when we are asleep, and much of the work of modern psychologists, such as Freud, is devoted to showing that we constantly have volitional (Lat. *volo*=wish) processes of which we are unconscious. The ' libido ' which now appears so prominently in psycho-analytical writings, is a name for this general striving activity, which throughout life is never suspended.

How this stream of striving proceeds in any individual depends partly on sensations impressed by the external world, but also partly on internal factors. Certain of the latter are of particular importance, because their character determines the direction of the stream. It is to these factors the terms *Instinct, Impulse, Interest, Need,* refer. Pleasantness and painfulness clearly play a great part in controlling our behaviour, and this pleasure-pain aspect of experience is what is generally spoken of as feeling-tone.

Consciousness. Where in such an account does consciousness (Lat. *conscio*=know) appear ? It cannot be too clearly realized that much of what is quite properly to be called mental activity is not conscious. Only some of the elements involved have the peculiar character which we name consciousness. But we should be careful when we use the term 'element'. A mental state is not built up of items as a wall is of bricks. This is an error which has long haunted psychology and is known as associationism or atomism. What were supposed to be the bricks were mental occurrences of two kinds, sensations and images. They have received a disproportionate amount of study because they are the mental events which are most easily introspected. Sensations—and in this statement we are adopting a highly controversial view, the alternatives to which are discussed in Chapter II—are happenings in the nervous system, due to stimuli from outside the body, *e.g.*, in vision, or to the stimulation of one part of the body by another. A toothache, or a colic, is the same in its mode of origin as the sensation obtained, *e.g.*, by clenching the fist. The importance of these sensations, due to the action of one part of the body on another, will be clear when we come to discuss *emotions*; and they have much bearing upon the growth of self-consciousness and of our knowledge of other minds.

It is obvious that not all effects of stimuli

are, or give rise to, conscious perceptions. What may be the difference between effects which give rise to consciousness and those which do not is a matter upon which little light has yet been thrown. Consciousness is supposed to be associated with the higher parts of the nervous system, the bringing in of these higher systems accompanying the act of *attending*. It is plain that attention may make conscious what has hitherto been present but unperceived. If we keep our eyes motionless, we can discover, by merely attending to the edges of the field of view, that we are all the time seeing far more than we are ordinarily conscious of seeing. Similarly with all our senses. Without changing anything in our stimulation we can bring into explicit awareness much that lies ordinarily outside it—*e.g.*, the feel of our clothing on the skin and the rhythmic tension and relaxation of our breathing. Thus at all times there is a large field of inattention (stimulation not attended to) which is affecting us without causing consciousness.

Images. The other kind of ' element ' which invites introspection is the *image*, the representative of perception which occurs without the stimulus required for the perception.

A great deal of work has been done on images since Galton's *Inquiry into Human Faculty* drew attention to the vast range of difference between individuals both as to the images they habitually employ, and as to their powers of forming imagery of any kind. To-day, however, psychologists of all schools lay less stress upon images as an essential feature of mental life ; and there are some, such as Professor Watson, in his *Behaviorism* (1925), who deny that any kind of imagery is necessary, or indeed occurs at all. There is also an interesting controversy as to how far thought can be conducted without it. But in most people all kinds of imagery undoubtedly occur—visual, auditory, tactual, olfactory, gustatory, motor, kinæs-thetic, thermal, and organic. In fact, it is possible to form images corresponding to every kind of sensation.

The reader should discuss imagery with his friends, getting them to describe what they see when they imagine, *e.g.*, a monkey riding a bicycle, and asking them to give the monkey a top hat with a red rosette, etc. He will find that they differ greatly both in the vividness of their imagery and in their power of controlling it. It seems likely that special powers of imagery in one direction or another are due in large part to early trends of interest ; and if, as seems probable, various abilities depend largely on these trends and the imagery to which they give rise, it should eventually be possible to avoid much disappointment and waste of time due to the later selection of unsuitable occupations.

These great differences between the types of imagery which are employed by different people raise a special problem, as to how far people with different imagery can be said to have the same thoughts. If my consciousness is filled, say, with mental pictures (visual images) and your consciousness is filled with the mental echoes of the sounds of words, how can we be said to have the same thoughts ? And yet there is plainly a sense in which people who use quite different images can be said truly to be in agreement, to be thinking similarly.

Ideas. This problem, which is very important both historically and theoretically, is the same as the old question, " What is an Idea ? " when this question is asked in Psychology. The full answer is very complicated, but an outline may be given which

shows how the difficulty we have raised,
which would result from an attempt to
identify ideas with images, may be avoided.

For this purpose we require the biological
notion of adaptation with which we began.
All thinking, all mental activity, occurs in
the course of adaptation. When we have
an image, the actual occurrence (which appears
to us as an image) is a step in an actual or
possible adaptation. It is a repetition of a
step in a previous adaptation, namely, that
which we made when we had the original
sensation of which the image is sometimes
said to be a copy.

An adaptation involves something to which
we are adapting. If, for instance, I am thinking of St Peter's by means of an image of
its dome, and you are thinking of it by
means of the words 'St Peter's', we shall
each be adapted to something. If this is
the same, then we can be said to be thinking
of the same thing, and so to be having the
same thoughts—*i.e.*, adaptations—the same
ideas, in spite of the difference in our imagery.
Thus an *idea* (an ambiguous word which is
synonymous with a 'representation', a 'conception', a 'concept', a 'notion', or a
'universal') is a way of thinking applicable to

something, and as is implied by the term
' adaptation ', all ' thought ' is determined by
the necessity of reacting to situations and
determines action of some kind or other.

Emotions. We may now, bearing in
mind this idea of adaptation, turn to the
active side of mental processes, to striving,
and consider instincts and the emotions.
The distinctive feature of emotional as opposed
to other experience is the presence of certain
organic sensations, due to physiological
changes in the internal organs of the body,
such as a quickened pulse and arrested
breathing. These, or images of them, give
their peculiar flavour to experiences such as
anger, fear, love, or wonder.

Instincts. But it must not be supposed
that these sensations are all that constitutes
such an emotion as anger. We have to
examine the causes to which the sensations
themselves are due. We then find that there
are apparently a small number of primitive
drives or inborn arrangements of the organism,
which lead it to respond to special situations
in a special manner. These are, or may give
rise to, the so-called *instincts*. Thus if a
jaguar rushes suddenly upon us, our instinctive adaptation takes the form of *flight*.

But to facilitate flight the internal conditions of the body (the heart-beat, the breathing, the glandular activities, etc.) are modified; and these modifications give rise to the sensational part of the emotions above indicated. In other words, we are sorry, as James put it, because we cry, rather than *vice versa*. But a fly in the eye will make that organ water, yet we do not necessarily experience grief. That is to say, it is only bodily sensations, instinctively originated, which constitute emotions, or 'affects', as they are often called by modern writers; and there is much more in an emotion than a mere organic disturbance. Some would maintain that emotions may accompany instincts even when not consciously experienced, but are "in the unconscious" to which we may now turn.

The Unconscious. The recognition, chiefly since the opening of the present century, that most of our mental life has not the character of consciousness, is responsible for much of the present popular interest in the subject. The laws of the interconnections of conscious 'elements' had been elaborately studied a hundred years ago by writers like Hartley, and already by the time of John Stuart Mill it seemed unlikely that much more could be added. Authorities like Bain were producing definitive treatises on the intellect and the emotions, and, though there were sporadic attempts to found a science of animal psychology, and laboratory methods were being developed, it hardly appeared possible to do more than put the finishing touches on so monumental a structure.

At this point morbid psychology, through the work of medical men and alienists, specialists in the treatment of those who are beside themselves (Lat. *alius* = other), began to force upon the attention of the official representatives of the science the necessity for fresh hypotheses.

As so often, advance was due to the fresh stimulus provided by strange occurrences for which accepted theories could suggest no explanation. Hypnotism, alternating personalities, automatic writing and psychical research, hysteria, phobias and neuroses in general, particularly those relating to sex, became the central points of interest. Resemblances between the phenomena of dreams and those of mental diseases led to a completely new account of what happens in the mind when conscious control is relaxed.

The facts thus brought to light show that only a small part of our mental life is under conscious control, *i.e.*, controlled by processes which are themselves conscious. This has emphasized the fact that consciousness is the exception rather than the rule in the processes studied by psychology. In dealing, however, with ' The Unconscious ' which is becoming too ready a resource in psychological difficulties, the first necessity is to decide precisely how we are going to use our language. Most discussions of the unconscious proceed as though there were two distinct realms, the conscious and the unconscious; as when it is said that what was in the unconscious can be brought into consciousness or what is conscious may be repressed into the unconscious. The mind is thus regarded as composed of separate strata, and in addition to the Unconscious we hear of the Sub-conscious, the Fore-conscious, and so forth. This metaphorical language is convenient for some purposes, but no clear understanding of the problems can be reached unless we are prepared to go behind such verbal devices.

Metaphors and Facts. The result of rash speculations on the contents of the Un-conscious has been a revival of almost mediæval views of 'possession'—whereby from time to time the personality is invaded and occupied by what amounts to a separate spirit.

Arising out of the metaphor of 'force' in physics we have an extensive metaphorical vocabulary of impulsions, resistances, impacts, pulls and pushes, which at a certain level of analysis have their usefulness, but are carefully excluded by the physicist from any exact statement. Similarly, we may use the metaphors of 'unconscious desires', 'the censor', 'repressed complexes', and we then get what is the usual psycho-analytic description of a dream. It is hardly necessary to point out that all this metaphorical language will vanish as the science advances. But just as the scaffolding erected by builders is often more interesting to the public than their final architectural achievements, so the psychology of desire and memory in its early stages has lent itself to a picturesque treatment which, now that its work has been done, can profitably be discarded.

With these general considerations before us we may come to grips with our subject by introducing the momentous problem of Mind and Body.

CHAPTER II

THE MIND AND THE BODY

Mind, Soul, and Spirit. Upon the most interesting of all questions, "What is the mind?" psychologists are as yet by no means agreed. And it is unlikely that any amount of mere discussion and argumentation will lead to agreement. More facts are needed, and time for a realization of the bearing of these facts upon the general problem. The question has not yet become, as it must if it is to be solved, a purely scientific matter. Men's prejudices, preferences, and desires still intervene to make cool judgment difficult.

It is usual in psychology to include under the term 'mind' what in ordinary speech would be regarded as special attributes relating not to thought alone, but to the 'emotions', the 'passions', the 'affections', the 'heart', to 'intuition', to the 'soul', and to the 'spirit'. Popular opinion often assumes that these things are distinct from mind, which is regarded as chiefly concerned with the intellect, and it is sometimes convenient to distinguish emotion and will as ' spiritual ', and thought or intellect as ' mental '. But all these, as we shall see in Chapter XI, are, of course, inseparable aspects of the same stream of activity.

Even psychologists, however, have felt that the too exclusive preoccupation of academic thinkers (such as Mill, Mach, Meinong, Moore, Marty, and Maier—to confine ourselves to one letter of the alphabet only) with intellectual analysis has unduly warped the subject, and that some term more comprehensive than ' mind ' might be desirable. The term ' psychical ', as applied to ' psychical development ', ' psychical qualities ', etc., has long been familiar, though the advance of Psychical Research, the study of supernormal mental phenomena, has tended to give it and particularly the word ' psychic ' a supernatural tinge.

But if we oppose the brain to the ' mind ' in its narrower sense, some more general term, the ' psyche ', would be opposed to the body, the ' soma ', as a whole ;   it need hardly be pointed out that an experience is not connected solely with the brain, for the stomach, and the solar and sympathetic ganglia (Chapter XIV), may be playing their part.

The Seven Theories. To approach psychology through the Body-Mind controversy is one of the best ways of going quickly to the heart of the matter. Many conflicting views are still held by thinkers whose opinions are worthy of respect and consideration. The number of theories theoretically possible as to the relations of mind and matter is, it may surprise the reader to learn, only seventeen, and the parent of many of them[1] slays six of his offspring in a single paragraph ; but of those which concern the psychologist only seven are of importance.

(1) MATERIALISM   AND   BEHAVIORISM. There is the view of the Behaviorists and the Materialists that what appears to be mental is in reality physiological processes. Thinking, for example, according to Professor Watson, is *sub-vocal talking* ; that is to say,

---

[1] C. D. Broad, *Mind and its Place in Nature* (1925), pp. 611-612. The same writer's *Scientific Thought* (1924) gives a good idea of the meticulous analysis to which our views of ' Nature ' must be subjected before the modern physicist can even approach the still more elusive complexities of ' Mind '. As regards the relative importance of the theories thus distinguished, however, the view adopted in the following pages differs considerably from that of Dr Broad.

C

silent internal discourse—very slight muscular movements in the organs of speech or elsewhere in the body. Mental events, on this view, simply do not exist. What has always been regarded as experience, as the working of the mind, is an illusion, like the malevolence attributed by the savage to a pistol. All that we do is to respond by activities of our muscles and glands to the situations which we encounter. The main motive of this school is a passionate desire to avoid all mention in psychology of anything inaccessible to standard methods of observation.

When Materialism is inverted we get the various forms of Spiritualism (philosophically termed Idealism) according to which matter is an illusion and the only ' reality ' is mental.

(2) ANIMISM AND INTERACTIONISM.   In vigorous opposition to the materialists are the Animists (Lat. *anima*=soul), of whom Professor McDougall is the most uncompromising. They maintain that whatever may be the status of these material phenomena, however far neurology may go in explaining the processes which occur in the body, none the less, there is a mind or soul also :   a spiritual thing utterly different in nature from the body, which *interacts* with the body,

being affected by it and likewise affecting it. The old view that the Conservation of Energy made this interaction impossible is now abandoned; but the nature of the interaction which occurs remains so obscure, owing to our ignorance both of mind and of body, that the doctrine is at present almost without significance.

Various hypotheses have been devised to avoid either of these opposed positions, to escape both Materialism and Animism. The most widely adopted is Parallelism.

(3) PSYCHO-NEURAL PARALLELISM. According to parallelists there is a mind quite distinct from the body, but mind and body do not influence each other in any degree or at any point. Instead, it is supposed that every event in the higher parts of the nervous system is accompanied by a mental event, and *vice versa*. The two streams, neural and mental, run parallel to each other, but in complete independence: like two clocks, back to back, keeping time. This is perhaps the safest view in psychology; on the other hand it does not fully satisfy many of its adherents.

(4) EPIPHENOMENALISM. Or again, mind might be a by-product, an epiphenomenon,

of neural processes, not reducible to such processes, but still quite unable to influence them. It would be like a phosphorescent glow due to the neural processes which would go on regardless of it ; or, to adopt a perhaps more appropriate metaphor, it would be like the light emitted by an arc-lamp as the current passes across the gap between the carbons. This view, associated with the name of T. H. Huxley, has lately receded in favour of

(5) THE DOUBLE ASPECT HYPOTHESIS. Both mind and brain might be equally real, neither reducible to the other, but each of them ' aspects ' of something else. Both what we experience—*i.e.*, our mental processes—and what others, if they could look into our heads, would observe, are on this view equally signs of more fundamental happenings. The very same event which *appears to me* as my thought would *appear to you*, if you could see it, as my nervous system in agitation. The evident disadvantage of such a double aspect theory is that the fundamental happenings are left in such obscurity. They would seem to be things we could know nothing about.

(6) NEUTRAL MONISM. To avoid such unknowables, a new suggestion has recently

been put forward by Bertrand Russell. Mind he reduces to sensations and images, and these are regarded as probably reducible to physiological events ; at the same time his treatment of matter, including the body, turns the universe into sensations and sensibilia—*i.e.*, possible sensations. Thus the two meet in *one* (Gk. *monos*=one) kind of neutral stuff, those changes in this stuff which follow psychological laws being mental, those which follow physical laws being physical. Much interest is certain to centre round this view, which is, however, far from representing a stable position.

It is fortunately not necessary for psychology to decide at the outset between these rival hypotheses. Almost all its results can be stated in terms of any of them with more or less trouble in different cases : and perhaps the most interesting point in the controversy is the extreme difficulty of finding any facts which might decide between them when apparent differences due to the prejudices which they invite have been eliminated. This circumstance has suggested a seventh view which is much akin to the Double Aspect theory and is gaining ground.

(7) THE DOUBLE LANGUAGE HYPOTHESIS regards neurology and psychology as being concerned with the very same facts, but concerned to describe them in two different languages.

Every remark in the one science can theoretically be translated into terms of the other. The two accounts deal not with different aspects of some further unknowable event, but with the very same event, which is known in two ways: directly. in introspection, or when we are or enjoy an experience ; indirectly, in neurology, when through the interpretation of signs we infer an event in the brain. As Professor Piéron in introducing his masterly survey of modern research, *Thought and the Brain*, admirably remarks :

" Whatever certain theorists may assert to the contrary, neurophysiology does undoubtedly often provide an adequate representation of the laws established by psychology ; the study of the functions of the brain frequently supplies satisfying explanations of psychological phenomena. In fact, we often pass from one form of representation—or rather, from one form of expression or language—to the other."

Many adherents of the Double Aspect formulation would probably subscribe to the Double Language view if they considered the alternative more closely. But a peculiar effort of the imagination is required before the idea becomes plausible. An experience and an agitation in the body seem so unlike one another that the suggestion that they are one and the same, and that the difference is merely in our mode of access to them, is often treated as outrageous. Yet it is the very uniqueness of experience which suggests this view; and those who dismiss its advocates as unable to appreciate the obvious fact that experience is unique are frequently unaware of the weight of considered opinion in favour of the linguistic solution. We approach all other happenings from without; but our experience is a happening in ourselves. Thus it should naturally seem to us totally distinct from the happenings which we observe through signs; and if, as this view holds, *experience* can be observed from without, it must be unrecognizable as an experience. The unlikeness, therefore, would only be an argument against treating the experience and the nervous disturbance as identical if the psychologist introspecting and the neurologist making his conjectures were using the same kind of observation.

Language itself (always awkward when things which have been traditionally regarded as different have to be identified) and the absence of parallel instances, which could be used as analogies, are further difficulties. Thus it is often objected that we can ask questions about the brain—its shape, for example—which we cannot ask about the mind. It is true that such questions at present sound awkward ; but, to take a rough parallel, we do not, if we are wise, conclude that because the remark, " Parliament is hungry," sounds awkward, Parliament must therefore consist of something other than the human beings who forthwith proceed to lunch.

Advantages of the Linguistic Solution. The Double Language view retains the advantages of the physical approach while avoiding its incompleteness ;   for on this view psychology is no more reduced to neurology than neurology is reduced to psychology.   Both remain indispensable parts of a complete account.   Introspection, metaphorically speaking, studies life from within, neurology from without.   Each account supplements the other. Thus the natural prejudices on both sides have less play, and are less offended by this theory than by any of the rival views. Those who resent a solution which would reduce all mental life to a mere play of brain processes, governed by laws into which such things as hopes, desires, purposes, and aspirations do not enter can find on careful consideration no ground for objection ; for neural laws would be a translation of just these kinds of things into terms of neural action. At the same time those who despair of any science whose methods and results do not admit of control and corroboration by the methods and results of the other sciences will find their demand met.

In any case, it is important to notice how intimately observation of bodily behaviour, together with inferences as to the working of the nervous system, are mingled in all our descriptions of the events in our lives with observations of our feelings, our thoughts, our interests, and the rest of our experiences. Our movements, etc., are public facts, our experiences are private. A complete account of a minute of any person's life would have to mention both public and private facts. Neither alone would be adequate. It is those who are most expert in inferring the one kind of fact from the other who succeed in the world. There is nothing so important as to be able to pass without mistake from observation of the behaviour of other people to conclusions about their thoughts, feelings, and intentions ;   and conversely to pass without mistake from our own private experiences to conclusions about the external events which are influencing us and about the state of our bodies.

Programme. This division between observations from within and from without, therefore, will guide us in the division of our subject-matter. And since the stock of common knowledge is far greater as regards internal observations than external, we will begin by describing in outline the part which is less familiar, namely the working of the nervous system so far as this concerns psychology :   the more familiar part may then be considered in a new light. Keeping to the standpoint of external observation, we shall sketch the growth of the mind from its earliest forms to its present development in man. When we have carried our neurological account as far as possible, we shall turn to the psychological account and describe the mind as it appears *from within*. Knowledge gained by either method will be found invaluable in the development of the other.

It is significant that so conservative an authority as Professor Lashley has recently warned his less critical colleagues that " psychology is to-day a more fundamental science than neurophysiology. By this I mean that the latter offers few principles from which we may predict or define the normal organization of behaviour, whereas the study of psychological processes furnishes a mass of factual material to which the laws of nervous action in behaviour must conform." Once again, then, if we are careful not to take the descriptive term too seriously, the proper study of mankind is " mind."

CHAPTER III

IMPULSE AND INHIBITION

The Action of Neurones. The body is a vast society of living cells, many hundreds of thousands of millions in number ; each of these cells has its special task, its contribution towards the activity of the whole society. Each, of whatever kind it may be, in skin or bone or muscle or gland, depends for its life upon the co-operation in numberless ways of other kinds of cells. But this co-operation does not come about of itself. Special arrangements are needed to adjust the different activities of separate groups of cells to one another ; and, what is equally important, to put the organism as a whole into adjustment with what is happening outside it. From minute to minute the situation in which we find ourselves changes ; we need to make suitable corresponding changes ourselves. Conversely, our own internal state changes and we need to make suitable changes in the situation. The principal agent whereby this is done is the nervous system.

The nervous system is itself made up of living cells which specialize as conductors, handing on disturbances which arise in one part of the body so that other parts of the body can deal with the situation. These cells (known as neurones) are of a fantastic variety of forms, but since they are all essentially conductors, they have a common plan. Each consists of a *cell-body*, which is as it were the commissariat department of the whole cell, looking after its nourishment and upkeep. It also provides for a varying number of prolongations, some of which are of great length, as when a neurone in the spinal cord sends an *axon* down to a toe muscle, while others (*dendrites*) communicate with structures at the same level.

When a stimulus is applied to one portion of the neurone a wave of change spreads through it at considerable speed (in man as high as 125 metres a second). This wave of change is handed on from neurone to neurone. They touch one another off as a series of fuses in contact might. The points of contact, known as synapses (Gk. *synapto*=join together), seem to act as valves: they let

the impulse pass in one direction only ;   it
is not allowed to return on its track.

The Conflict of Impulses. The central
problem is this—How does it happen that
an impulse takes one path on a given occasion
and not another ? To consider it we need a
clear idea of the system as a whole (cf. Fig. I)
and of the broad outlines of its working.

In the first place, it is an extraordinarily
unified system ; its various parts and their
separate activities are interdependent in the
highest degree. This must obviously be the
case in an organ whose job is to *integrate* the
body, to unite its activities into orderly
co-operative behaviour. But the rule that
what is happening in any one part of the
nervous system depends upon what is happening elsewhere holds good throughout, and
we must strenuously resist the temptation to
regard any particular impulse as an isolated
happening.

If a wasp stings my finger I usually take
the finger away from it, and it is tempting
to analyse this impulse as though the rest
of the goings-on in my nervous system were
irrelevant. But if I were hanging over a
precipice by that hand alone I should not
try to wave it about, however busy the wasp

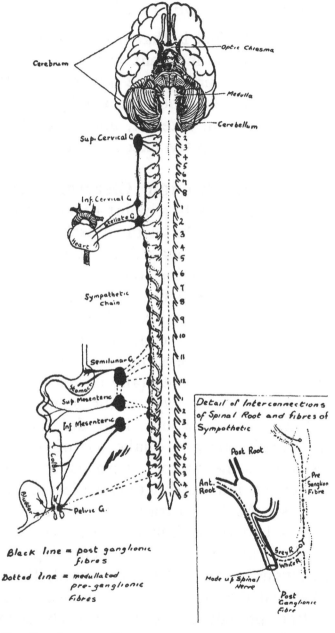

FIG. I.—GENERAL DIAGRAM OF THE NERVOUS SYSTEM.
Showing the relationship of the central nervous system to the
sympathetic.

might be. The fact is that even the impulses which seem most insistent and independent have merely a precedence *allowed* by the others. They take their course by consent and in the general interest, and may, if the situation is sufficiently exceptional, be overruled.

Adjustment through Clearing-houses. The instance suggests a point of view which is illuminating. The arm muscles of the wasp's victim are engaged for the moment in the task of holding on. A special set of neurones (motor neurones) running *down* to them from the spinal cord is keeping them in the right state of contraction. But the sting of the wasp sets up an agitation in another set of neurones (afferent or sensory neurones) which run *up* to the spinal cord, and this agitation would, if it did not find them already engaged, make use of some of those very same motor neurones to throw the muscles into a different series of contractions. At the entrance to these motor neurones two rival claimants for the use of them have arisen. Now the central part of the nervous system (the spinal cord, that is to say, and the brain) is an arrangement for adjusting precedences between such claims in view of the whole relevant situation. The motor neurone, or the similar apparatus in the case of a gland, is therefore sometimes called the " final common path ". It is an apparatus at the disposal of an immense number of impulses from different sources, some of which can use it together while others obviously can only use it in turn. In between the sources of these impulses and the motor apparatus intervenes tier after tier of clearing-houses sorting out rival claims, combining some, holding up others, according to the complexity of the relevant situation. The situation relevant to the way we breathe, for example, is fairly simple. The main factors are the state of the atmosphere and of the blood and the position of the body. So the adjustment of the various claims can ordinarily be left to the more lowly centres as a routine business. But for the singer and the Everest climber the matter is more complicated ; higher-level clearing-houses have to take charge, and since these higher centres are less used to the business, a learning process is required.

The Importance of the Head. The highest centres are those which have to take note of the widest and most intricate situations and to order the largest and most varied sets of claims. For reasons which are clear enough in outline they lie in the head—in the ' cerebrum ' and ' cerebellum '.

The exact topographical site of the various orders of clearing-houses which occur in the brain (as to which a good deal is beginning to be known) is of no general importance for psychology. An idea of some of the areas which are known to be concerned with special functions can be gathered from Fig. II. It is the scheme of their relations to one another that matters. Each clearing-house is a fairly extensive region where innumerable cell-bodies with their dendrites and axons, interlacing and criss-crossing in every direction in a tangle of incredible complexity, are massed together. Cell-bodies and dendrites are gray, axons are white in appearance ; hence the name ' gray cells ' or ' gray matter ' for those parts of the brain in which the most complex transactions take place. The most accessible region, stretching over the surface like the peel of an orange, is known as the cortex. We need not enter into further detail here, for the reader will find a clear account of the nervous system in *The A B C of the Nerves*, by Professor D. F. Fraser

Harris, uniform with the present volume.

Inhibition. The exact way in which neurones interact is still largely a matter of speculation. What little we know of them

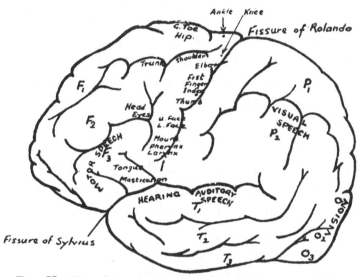

FIG. II.—THE LOCALIZATION OF FUNCTION IN THE BRAIN
(*Seen from the left side*).

The area thickly spotted with names just in front of the Rolandic fissure is the *motor* area, and if it is electrically stimulated ' voluntary' movements of the parts indicated occur. The corresponding areas on the other side of the fissure are *reception* centres for touch sensations from the same parts. The visual reception area is at the extreme back of the brain. Between this and the tongue area lie, with innumerable others, the association centres for reading.

comes chiefly from experiments upon what are referred to as ' spinal' reflexes. When the spinal cord is severed from the brain its operations are no longer controlled by the

higher clearing-houses, and a great simplifica-
tion results ; further, as there is clear evidence
to show, consciousness, including pain, for
the parts thus cut off, no longer occurs.   It
is then possible to elicit movements, say of
the leg, by simple stimuli in a very uniform
manner.   By combining stimuli and noting
the responses, something of the ways in which
impulses combine or interfere with one another
can be made out.

In every movement the motor neurones
concerned have to see that one set of muscles
contracts and the opposite set relaxes.   In
other words, introducing an important technical term for an idea which is fundamental
in psychology, one set of muscles is excited
and the other set is *inhibited* (Lat. *inhibeo*
=check.)   Various theories have been put
forward to account for the inhibition of
impulses.   The latest is in terms of that
neuro-muscular attunement with which we
shall be concerned in the next Chapter,
where it helps us to understand some of the
workings of memory.   Needless to say, whatever account of inhibition is ultimately
accepted it will be highly complicated.

One special feature, which no theory yet
satisfactorily explains, is probably of con-

siderable psychological importance. This is the ' rebound ', following inhibition, which is often experimentally discoverable. The inhibited activity starts again with renewed vigour when the inhibition is removed. Whether this is always so cannot at present be decided, but there are many obvious facts in everybody's experience which suggest that it may be very general ; ˙the increased vigour of a ' temptation ', for example, which is only momentarily quashed, and many of the phenomena unearthed by psycho-analysis.

CHAPTER IV

HOW THE BRAIN WORKS

The Relation of Higher and Lower Levels. We have now to consider how the various higher and lower-level clearing-houses in the nervous system are related to one another. Instead, however, of starting with one particular stimulus and asking how it comes to arouse a particular response, we must begin, as psychologists, with the total situation in which the body finds itself. Of the innumerable impulses which are coming in from the greater number of our sense organs all the while, only a small proportion can ultimately reach the final common paths, the motor neurones which excite the muscles. But very many which themselves play no final part have yet, at one level or another, a say in what finally shall take place ; typically by barring out other impulses which otherwise would get through. And only a small proportion of these ultimately give rise to consciousness in the form of mediating the individual's *awareness* of some part of the situation. A process of selection takes place quite early in the afferent (incoming) course of the impulse. Further, a set of excitations which in themselves would each be unnoticed and have no central effects may, if they happen to come together in a certain pattern, get through and take effect at once ; for example, a set of black and yellow streaks in the landscape when, and only when, coiled upon one another in the rattlesnake fashion, or a set of sounds in an otherwise unnoticed hubbub if they happen to be arranged in the pattern of our own name.

Reception Centres. Thus the notion of *reception centres* which act as a kind of selective sieve becomes necessary ; and the actual location of some of these centres in the cerebral cortex has been discovered. Here a preliminary sorting out occurs. For example, other things being equal, a stimulus which is unlike its neighbours has a better chance of getting through, and certain kinds of impulses have almost invariable precedence. Again impulses arising from stimuli harmful to the skin override all others. But hard upon this simpler kind of sorting out there follows

a more complicated task—that of responding
to certain patterns, as with the snake or the
name, and not to others.   The reception
apparatus recognizes some patterns just as
a lock ' recognizes ' its key. It is not difficult
to imagine this being done by a system of
neurones which discharge other systems only
when excited together or in a certain order.
But the fact that we ' recognize ' our names
when spoken by very different voices raises
a great difficulty which we shall note again
in our chapter on Perception.

Co-ordination Centres. The reception
centres are in close connection then with
sensory co-ordination centres, as these arrangements which pick out patterns among incoming impulses are called. Certain injuries,
it is found, may incapacitate the co-ordination centres without disturbing the receptive
centres. In such a case there might be nothing
detectably wrong with the patient's vision,
for example, in itself ; he would not be blind,
he would merely not recognize anything he
saw.

On the inner side of the sensory co-ordination centres there will be many further centres
which carry out the same kind of transactions
as the co-ordination centres ; only this time

with the products of the co-ordination centres and not with original impulses from the sense organs. We may call these higher clearing-houses the *association areas*.

Expectation. So far we have been tracing the march of the armies of impulses inwards, but by the time the association centres are in play there may be corresponding movements outwards, from higher centres to lower, from association centres to sensory co-ordination centres. The influence of expectation on perception is clear evidence for this. If we are expecting a certain person to appear in the distance we are extremely likely to mistake other people for her. Now an expectation in such a case involves a special setting of a co-ordination centre brought about by an association centre, a certain preparedness to pick out one pattern rather than others. What we know from within as 'attention' is accompanied by a heightening of tone. An impulse or influence from above alters the lock, so that the impulses coming in from the receptive centre may more easily turn it.

We must think, then, of these tides of impulses as having eddies, through which what has already reached the centres controls what is still coming in. There will be circuits of this kind not only from association centres to co-ordination centres, but from higher to lower association centres. A typical case is the influence exercised by a general conception (which is the activity of an association centre of relatively high level) upon the particular instances of experience which can be brought under it. When we know that a thunderstorm is an electrical phenomenon, it is no longer quite so easy to regard it as a judgment upon our actions. Even the most intricate intellectual play of ideas—the mastering of a psychological theory, for example—may be imagined as consisting of the same kind of transactions as those of the co-ordination centres and the reflex centres of the spinal cord, but carried out at higher levels and perhaps of even greater complexity.

The Influence of the Past. In one respect which has not yet been mentioned the complexity is certainly greater. The higher we go in the nervous system the more definite and more subtle the influence of the past becomes.

What exactly memory may be in terms of the nervous system is a problem which is still a very long way from solution. It is better perhaps to speak of *retention* than memory, for memory may mean either recollection (I have a memory of The Great Boer War) or that I now can do something (*e.g.*, swim) which I could not do if I had not done it before. The second is the sense in which retention is used. The first (recollection) is a special instance of the working of retention.

Retention is already active at the level of the sensory co-ordination centres; it is essentially a matter of the repetition of certain co-ordinations even when the circumstances are no longer the same. It shows itself in two ways at every stage of co-ordination right up to the highest levels.

Retention and the Conditioned Reflex. The response on repetition may become quicker, smoother, more perfect of its kind, as we see happening in the formation of *habits;* or it may dispense with some part of the stimulation which was originally necessary, as we see most clearly in the formation of what are known as *conditioned* reflexes. Usually the two effects of retentiveness go together.

When two impulses have co-operated to produce a certain response it is found that after a sufficient number of repetitions one of them alone may bring it about, though formerly inadequate by itself. Such a response is said to be ' conditioned '; a new stimulus has been substituted for the old, and the response now occurs under new conditions. In man very few repetitions may be sufficient ; but after infancy all his reactions are made to such complicated situations that it is far easier to study conditioned responses in animals. Even here, however, the most elaborate precautions are required to exclude disturbing factors.

The fundamental work on this subject has been done by Pavlov and his assistants in Leningrad, and the results already attained seem likely to be of the utmost assistance to psychology. They are the foundation of the theories of the Behaviorist School to which we devote a special chapter. Pavlov has found it best to work with one particular response. A dog secretes saliva when given food. It is his first step towards digesting it. Now all through the evolution of the dog (the same is true of man) he has been constantly on the lookout for signs of food. He is thus specially prepared for all kinds of different stimuli to become connected in his association centres with the presence of food. This gives the investigator his opportunity.

Every time food is put before the dog a particular note, for example, is sounded. After a certain number of repetitions of this combination the note is sounded alone. The

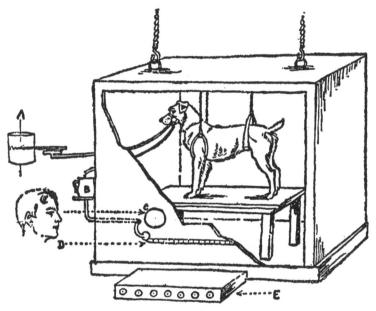

Fig. III.—Pavlov's Dog.

A. Revolving drum for recording rate of secretion of saliva.
B. Vessel for receiving salivary secretion.
C. Observation window or periscope for observing the dog.
D. Graduated scale to measure quantity of salivary secretion.
E. Electric contacts to set source of stimulus in operation.

dog's mouth waters. A conditioned reflex has been established. It may be added that the dog does not seem to be averse from this experiment, and jumps of his own accord on to the table where he appears in Fig. III.

By this method many very remarkable phenomena have been brought to light.

Not only is the dog's discrimination of pure tones vastly superior to that of the best human musicians, but it is significant that neurasthenia may result if the dog is persistently given too difficult a task. If, for example, he is forced to attempt a discrimination between shapes which are too similar for him, he little by little loses all his previously acquired conditioned reflexes. He even fails in the end to discriminate between what is edible and what is not. At the same time he becomes quarrelsome, dirty, and unmanageable, howls at the moon and finally ends up in a state of general incompetence. A prolonged rest cure at the farm is needed to restore him to his former good-tempered sanity. The general bearing of these results, when they are explained, upon human psychology is likely to be immense. But we must return to the problem presented by the simplest case of conditioning.

The point to note is that here we have a response, the watering of the dog's mouth, which would not have occurred if the conditioned stimulus (the note) and the unconditioned stimulus (the food) had not been

combined in the comparatively remote past.
The past conjunction has left some effect
in the dog's nervous system through which
the note alone produces the response which
formerly required the presence of the food.
How are we to conceive this effect?

It used to be supposed that images could
be stored up in the cells of the brain, and
their co-operation was assumed to settle the
problem. But an image is a process, a
transaction, just as much as a perception;
it is a happening. And there is every reason
to suppose that images only differ from the
actual experiences by being aroused not
through incoming impulses from the receptive
centres but through impulses of central origin.
We call them images because they correspond to perceptions. They are due in some
way to persistent effects (called by Semon
'engrams,' but the more usual term in
psychology is 'disposition' or 'trace')
left behind by perceptions, but they are not,
themselves, those effects. What lasts is not
the image, but as Hering said, " the peculiar
attunement (*Stimmung*) of the nervous substance in virtue of which it will give out
to-day the same note that it gave out yesterday, if the strings be touched aright "

Another explanation in terms of a deepening of nervous channels may be much more on the right lines.   But we must take account of the end-state of the whole process, the success or failure at the point which matters to the animal, if we are to explain the variations in the means by which it is brought about.   In other words, all behaviour is purposive, though it may often be so ill directed, incomplete, and confused that we cannot pick out the purpose.   The mainspring of these conditioned reflexes is the dog's need for food.   If we leave this out of consideration we shall naturally find the facts difficult to explain.

Success as Establishing Attunement. Neither the impulses from the note nor those from the food come into an indifferent brain. The latter find a centre already tuned for them by the emptiness of the dog's viscera. The impulses from the note reach this centre —and they must reach many other centres besides.   The fact to be explained is that after a certain number of conjunctions of note-impulses with food-impulses, the centre discharges on the arrival of the note-impulses alone.   We must remember that practically any stimulus in place of a note can be conditioned in the same fashion. Even a painful stimulus can. All symptoms of fright or pain cease and a severe pinch or bruise merely causes abundant salivation. Nothing brings out the interdependence of the processes in the brain better than this astonishing fact. Whatever sensory stimulus—whether from a colour, a noise, a touch, an electric shock, or what not—immediately precedes the giving of the food, the impulse it arouses comes to discharge the centre in place of the food-impulse, given sufficient repetition.

The difficulty of understanding how this happens is due to thinking of the centre in two phases only—as it is when the note-impulse reaches it, and as it is when the food-impulse causes it to discharge. Instead, we must think of it in four phases—

(1) as it is when played upon by hunger-impulses before the note-impulse comes in,

(2) as it is when this impulse has altered it,

(3) as it is when the food-impulse discharges it,

(4) as it is when the consequences of the arrival of the food in the stomach are playing upon it.

E

This last seems to be the decisive phase in tuning the centre to discharge henceforward on the mere arrival of the note-impulse. We may suppose that the food- and note-impulses together leave the neurones of the centre in a peculiar state which lasts for a little while, and that the incoming of the impulses from the stomach fixes this state. Next time the note-impulse comes in it finds the centre still tuned in the same way—tuned, that is, to be discharged either by the note or by the food, and the centre discharges. In what this particular tuning consists is the great unsolved mystery of learning.

The most modern authorities are suggesting that the theory of the conditioned reflex has temporarily served its purpose, and though invaluable at a certain stage as an introduction, it may now be a barrier to fresh hypotheses. Recent work by Lashley[1] and others has tended to confirm the view that learning is a function of the total brain, which may explain the differences in the number of lessons required. Thus, a dog or a rat may need twenty or thirty, but in man, mastery

---

[1] "The cortex seems to provide a sort of generalized framework to which single reactions conform spontaneously as the words fall into the grammatical form of a language."—K. S. Lashley, " Basic neural mechanisms in behavior," *Psychological Review*, January, 1930, page 18.

can often be achieved at one stroke. Similarly, the time the fixation lasts varies greatly. In the dog, if we do not give him the note too often without the food, or otherwise bring in inhibitions, it lasts indefinitely, as it does in man. In the cockroach it seems to last at most half an hour. The memory of the cockroach is not very tenacious.

We can now see how it is that if we sound the note too often without food, we break down the conditioned reflex. The tides of impulses (phase 4) which come to the centre after salivation, from an empty stomach or a full, are very different; the tuning there, instead of being fixed, is changed. The note henceforth, instead of exciting the final common path, now inhibits it.

We have lingered somewhat over these intricacies, so that the reader may take stock of the difficulties; and also that he may realize why the physiological explanation of the brain's activities does not stand or fall with the success or failure of any one particular theory. There is still much work to be done in the physiological laboratory whose results will undoubtedly have a direct bearing on these problems. The main attack has not yet been made. The work so far done amounts to 'getting the guns into position' for that attack. So that to assume special 'psychical' agents, or to maintain that the working of the mind is beyond the scope of any possible physiological explanation, would be a rash procedure for a psychologist to-day.

CHAPTER V

PURPOSE AND INTEREST

Purpose and Foresight. There is another important reason for looking rather closely into the nervous mechanism of retention. Only so can we see its close connection with the *purposive* character of behaviour. An activity is said to be purposive when the result which it is going to produce seems to influence its course ; that is to say, when what is about to happen seems to be directing and controlling what is already happening. This kind of apparent causation by what does not yet exist, by the end or goal of an activity, is known in philosophical language as teleology and has always seemed a very mysterious affair. Many thinkers have regarded it as necessarily involving ' foresight ', meaning thereby something which no physical or physiological processes, however intricate, can explain. And unless we have an adequate conception of these intricacies, and especially of the ways in which retention complicates them, this view is very difficult to avoid. For this apparent foresight is entirely due to retention. It is due to the ways in which the effects of past activities control the present.

When it seems that we are being influenced by what is about to happen, by the results to come from what we are doing, we are really being influenced by the lingering effects of what has happened on former occasions in similar situations. And we are constantly being so influenced; in fact, nothing that we do is immune from the influence of similar situations in our past or that of an ancestor. So it is perfectly correct to say that all our behaviour has the peculiar character of purposiveness, a character not possessed by such physical processes as are involved when stones fall or clouds form or seas foam. But we should realize that this purposiveness is a physiological characteristic, that it is due to retention in living tissues and pre-eminently in the living systems which form the higher nervous centres. Physiological processes are, in the opinion of the most circumspect authorities, merely extremely complicated physical processes. The more complex systems which make up living tissue naturally behave in more complicated ways than the similar systems of physics.

Retention and Attunement. We take retention then as a fundamental fact in the working of the brain. It does not necessarily involve any storing up of impressions or images, or any laying down or scouring out of new paths or channels. To say that the brain retains a response is to say that certain stimuli may find it in the state of attunement in which that response left it, and that therefore if the situation recurs it will respond in the same way. This, of course, does not bar out the possibility of persistent modifications.

Recognition. So far we have discussed retention only as it appears in the simplest form of conditioned reflex. We shall see how universal the influence of the past upon the present is if we reflect upon some of the less simple forms. Consider the sensory co-ordination centres which we discussed above, and the way in which they pick certain patterns out of the welter of incoming impulses. The centre by which we recognize a series of sounds as being a certain tune is a good example. The first time this series of impulses comes into the centre we do not, of course, recognize it. But, since we have presumably heard other tunes before, it does not find the centre unprepared, and we have probably heard the same notes before. Each note has its own special effect upon the centre and is handed on as a special set of impulses different from those due to any other note. Further, each note leaves the centre ready to deal with some notes better than with others. As the tune proceeds a cycle of operations takes place in the centre, easier for some people than for others (what is called 'a good musical ear' is really a good centre) and easier if the tune is of a familiar kind, and if the transactions required in passing from note to note are fairly simple. Quite early on, after two or three notes perhaps, back into the centre come the consequences of the passing through of these notes. Every impulse that the centre hands on has a widespread reverberation all over the body, and the effects of these reverbera-tions come back to the centre and take a share in handling the following notes. This is why the earlier notes seem to make so much difference to the later ones. The later notes have actually to be handled differently by the centre because of the effects of the earlier. Finally the tune is completed, the last of the reverberation effects comes in and the centre is left more or less set for the handling of this tune in future, according as these reverberations are more or less satisfying to the whole organism. The process is quite parallel to that in Pavlov's dog.

When the tune is heard again and recognized, it is not in the least necessary, as everyone knows, to recollect the occasion on which it was formerly heard. All that is involved in mere recognition is that the centre is, on the second occasion, after the first few notes, set ready for the rest of the transaction. On the second occasion not only are the later notes influenced by the earlier, but also the earlier by the later; to put it more accurately, they are influenced by the still enduring effects of the notes which followed on the former occasion. This explains why a tune, though recognized as the same, yet often sounds very different on repetition, and why it is so easy to hear some tunes too often.

Interest and the Selection of Patterns. All recognition of other people, of our own name, of words, of places, of tables and chairs, of moods and emotions, of situations large or small, part or whole, is done in this fashion. The plan of the universe as we see it is the plan of the persistent accords in our nervous centres, the plan of the patterns by which we handle our stimulation. And as our instances have brought out, these patterns depend not only upon what is given in stimulation to our sense organs, but still more upon the relative satisfaction to us as integral individuals of picking out one pattern rather than another. The universe may be, and probably is, shouting at us all the time the clearest and most unmistakable news. Perhaps news which in the long run might be of overwhelming importance to our welfare. But if the immediate consequence of picking out the pattern of these ' messages ' is uncomfortable, or if it involves ceasing to pick out a pattern which suits us, we shall not hear them. As Professor Thurstone puts it, " while walking to your office . . . most of the signs, stores, vehicles, and people are indifferent stimuli which are not even perceived because you do not identify them with your purpose ".[1]

---

[1] *The Nature of Intelligence* (1924), p. 9.

The world as we ordinarily regard it, the world of roads, gardens, motor cars, noises, colours, bodies, and even of brains, is the indirect reflexion of our interests, since it is these which ultimately pick out the groups of stimuli which we treat as single things.

Hence it is that the conceptions even of homely and familiar objects—the wood in the grate, the wine in the wood, the billiard table, or the pussycat—entertained by people of different interests can vary so immensely. The accounts given of the wine by the chemist and the connoisseur are far removed.   The ordinary man is satisfied with an idea of a cannon which the physicist (as a physicist, not as a billiard-player) rejects *in toto*.   And how the physiologist regards the cat may be gathered to some extent from these pages.   The problem of picking and choosing among these points of view—which patterns to select—cannot be avoided by a psychologist. And he is, or should be, the man of all men who is best placed for considering it, since it is his job to study this choice between patterns and also the factors by which it is controlled.

In actual fact we pick out the pattern which best fits in with the dominant activity.

Pavlov's dogs pick out the note and treat it as a signal for salivation because food-seeking is their dominant activity. The errand boy picks up the tune because whistling is his. The physicist at the billiard-table discards all thoughts of electrons because pocketing the white is his main aim for the moment.

But, to return, what are these dominant activities, these purposes, these interests, which pick and choose among possible patterns ? Are they, too, conceivable in terms of the nervous system or have we here at last to abandon physiology and introduce something not of a physical order, in the form of psychic urges, instincts, wants, desires, strivings, an *élan vital* or a *libido*? Can these, too, be brought under our scheme of connected brain centres influencing one another and handing on impulses to one another, forwards and by backwash ? And lastly how do these interests, besides selecting what shall come in, also decide what goes out, and how do they translate the inner swirl of impulses into overt action ?

If we compare the body to a self-directing and self-regulating machine, however inappropriate from some points of view the comparison may be, we shall at least be reminded that, like an engine, it needs fuel. It uses up its supplies of energy and has to get more. Further, and here it differs from those simple physical systems we call engines, it dies unless it subdivides from time to time. In lowly animals the subdivision is simple ; in man it is complex and involves endless to-do. Again, man is a social animal. He cannot get on by himself and has to live in a herd. This also involves a vast ramification of consequences among which speech, sanitation, war, and the great majority of mental diseases are examples. We might go on extending the list of man's needs. Food and sex are the original roots of a good many of them, but there are probably others, as we shall see in Chapter VII.

Man's Fundamental Needs. A Need is an internal disequilibrium. If it continues unappeased the efficiency of the organism often declines. The three needs we have mentioned, food, sex, and society, are apt to be fatal unless supplied. Reproduction as a way of escape from death strikes the ordinary man as unsatisfying—but from the point of view of the biologist a man may be said to live on in his offspring. Deprived of society, the infant only lives a few hours, the child a few days, and the adult is rapidly impaired in a number of ways.

On primitive needs derivative needs become grafted. For example, food-seeking, except for a very few fortunates, involves locomotion. Now unless the locomotor apparatus is employed a detrimental condition arises, so that even persons who are regularly fed by others find they have to take exercise. A derivative need arises. In general, though there are exceptions, the possession of a capacity involves a need to employ it. This is more obviously so when the capacity has developed special structures in the body—noteworthy biceps, for example : the sad state of the retired boxer or oarsman is frequently remarked. Where mental capacities are in question there is more doubt. The need of the mathematician to keep up his studies, or of the stamp-collector to go on collecting, is less certain. Even here it will perhaps be agreed that, other things being equal, if no other interests can be found, they will be well advised to continue.

Another way in which needs ramify involves the principle of the conditioned reflex again. If I continually drink tea while I

am working I may find in time that I need
tea in order to work. The centres involved
have become tuned to work best in the tea-
intoxication condition. Such drug addictions
are a very clear example of acquired needs.
My state, however, when deprived of tea is
not of necessity detrimental to all my activities,
but only detrimental to the work.

We all suffer from innumerable parasitic
and conditioned needs of this kind. The
lecturer who cannot get on unless he fidgets
with the chalk, the dandy who cannot shine
in conversation unless his attire is elegant,
are obvious instances. The great Kant was
not at his best unless his gaze was fixed upon
a certain tower across the way ; in the course
of years a neighbour's tree grew up to inter-
cept this vision ;   the owner had to cut it
down before the Critical Philosophy could
proceed.

Fixations.   A very important group of
these conditioned needs are what the psycho-
analysts call fixations. A child whose tender-
ness and affection have for a long time been
centred exclusively on its mother often finds
it difficult to feel these emotions towards
anyone who does not resemble the mother in
certain respects. Many other instances from

the pathology of the mind will arise for consideration later. We have said enough to make plain how universally operative conditioned needs are, and can pass to the problem of interests.

The Nature of Interest. An interest is an activity set going and maintained by a need. There is no mystery (as opposed to intricacy) about the way in which the need provokes the activity. The disequilibrium which is the need fires volleys of impulses into the centres, and their response to this bombardment is the activity. They respond when they can. But the rest of the situation has to be fitting. We often have intense needs about which nothing can be done. We can then only wait for a change, and when the change comes, the activity starts in what seems an entirely spontaneous fashion. Our interest leaps to life, as we say. But more than a mere need is required before an interest develops. There must also be the nervous organization necessary in order to translate the need into activity. A man in a coma is in a desperate state of need, but he shows the minimum of interest.

We should be on our guard constantly as to how we use quantitative terms in speaking of interest. Moreover, a heightening of one interest is very often accompanied by a general heightening and widening all round. The Napoleons, the Goethes, and the Newtons, the men of the most intense interests, are commonly also the men with the most quick and varied simultaneous interests. The theory of the central reservoir is too crude. It reaches its highest absurdities in the hands of some psycho-analysts who are in the habit of asking where the *libido* has gone whenever an interest lapses. We can avoid these mistakes best by remembering that interest is not something additional to or behind activity, but just the activity itself.

Discrimination. Width, variety, and keenness of interests are marks of the superior mind because they are signs that in one respect at least the nervous system is well organized. But they may be accompanied by extreme stupidity. Sensitiveness as well as interest is necessary. Interest is a matter of the excitability of the centres concerned. Sensitiveness has to do with the delicacy and plasticity of their tuning. The sensitive man is he who discriminates when he is interested. The stupid man is he who does not; and discriminating is simply varying

F

the response as the situation varies. Since it is essentially plasticity of tuning, it is closely connected with retention. The discriminating are those who retain the relevant effects of past experience. Too intense an interest seems often to hinder discrimination. We get ' excited ', as we say, and no longer know what we are doing.

The Initiation of Action. The arrangements by which activity in the nervous system is translated into bodily action through the outgoing (efferent) nerve paths are very similar to those by which impulses from the sense organs are sorted, co-ordinated, and associated in the incoming (afferent) path. The association centres discharge into certain incito-motor centres which are among the best known regions of the cortex of the brain. These lie in a band roughly from ear to ear over the top of the head. If we give them a mild electric shock, as has been done by Dr. Harvey Cushing with the consent of a patient, the subject moves his limbs and does so with a full sense that he is voluntarily performing the action. This is quite different from the effect of stimulating the motor nerves in the spinal cord, or nearer still to the muscle. Then the patient merely

feels his limb contract involuntarily. The
bearing of these facts on the question of the
Will is obvious.

When we remember that every time we
move an arm or turn the head when walking,
hundreds of other muscles must make com-
pensating movements or we shall fall over,
it is easy to see that special co-ordinating
arrangements are required. Even more complicated reflex co-ordinations maintain, whenever possible, our orientation.

The remaining transactions of the nervous
system, notably those involved in pleasure and
pain, in reasoning, and in the phenomena of
deliberation, resolve, belief, prejudice, and
suggestion will be discussed at a later stage
when the introspective account of the mind
is before us. Emotion will also be treated
separately, and this account of the incomings
and outgoings of the central nervous system
is thus not complicated by a discussion of
that other nervous system known as the
involuntary or sympathetic (autonomic) which
is essentially concerned with our vegetative
life.

CHAPTER VI

THE GROWTH OF THE MIND IN ANIMALS

The Comparative Method. There are two ways of tracing the growth of the mind. We can take a series of animals from various levels of the biological scale and compare their behaviour, making cautious guesses at the kinds of experience which are likely to accompany it. Or we can study the development of behaviour and experience in the child as he grows up to manhood, supplementing this by comparisons between individuals who more or less perfectly achieve maturity. Both methods are instructive and the first naturally leads on to the second, since the most accomplished animals—chimpanzees and gorillas for example—seem, except as regards language, to reach and to stop short at about the stage at which a bright three-year-old child begins. Moreover, by studying animal behaviour we are likely to avoid some of the errors which a too exclusive

74

preoccupation with the child's mental life, as seen through its effects upon that of the adult, may introduce. The theories of psychoanalysis are peculiarly exposed to this danger.

Much of the difficulty of psychology has in fact arisen through studying mind in its most complex form in man. The minds of animals are much simpler than those of men, and, though more difficult to observe, are more easily understood when once satisfactory observations have been made. Even very lowly organisms such as *Amœba* display behaviour which to some has seemed to indicate a rudimentary mind. But in animals with a nervous system we are on firmer ground, and it would be strange if a study of their behaviour did not throw light upon our own. Man has developed certain of their capacities to an incomparable height, but though his activities are more complicated, they are still the same in essence.

The Nature of Instincts. Ants and bees have always been recognized as offering supreme examples of instinctive behaviour, and the notion of an instinct is fundamental to psychology. To understand what an instinct is we need the notion of heredity. Every living creature begins life with a congenital make-up, a set of innate arrangements for coping with the situations in which it finds itself. In the insects, which usually have to fend for themselves from the first, these arrangements include innate neural tunings (dispositions as they are called) through which a particular situation, a particular set of stimuli, leads to a particular kind of response, sometimes extraordinarily definite, complex, and appropriate.[1] This activity, which needs no learning and has no previous history, is said to be instinctive. And each well-marked kind of response corresponding to a well-marked kind of need and situation is called an *instinct*. There is no reason to suppose that instincts differ in any respect from other non-instinctive activities, except in being due to innate arrangements in the nervous system and not to arrangements which have been formed in the course of the vicissitudes of the individual's life. It is important not to regard an instinct as a peculiar kind of supernatural

---

[1] The fact that many eminent biologists are fully aware of the bearing of their material on general psychology, has added greatly to the value of their contributions of recent years. Bugnion's *The Origin of Instinct* (1927), Wheeler's *The Social Instincts* (1928), and Rabaud's *How Animals find their way about* (1928), are models of exposition and method alike.

force or wisdom. It is no more mysterious though no less, than any other of the animal's activities.

Instincts are not necessarily immutable. The nervous arrangements on which they depend are modifiable in greater or less degree. Wasps, for example, will enlarge the entrance to their nests when trial has shown that a spider cannot be dragged in, and ants which have been tricked into leaping from an eminence into vinegar refuse in the future, for a while at least, to take similar leaps. That is to say, they show evidence of having 'learned by experience'. Their behaviour, instead of being governed solely by innate arrangements in their nervous systems, is modified by their own individual experience. It becomes a blend, in other words, of instinctive and 'intelligent' behaviour. But if we pass from the insects to the vertebrates we find that this new factor of 'intelligence' increases immensely. It is comparatively powerless in the insect and its effects are brief. The cockroach, as we saw, forgets its lessons in half an hour, the elderly ant and the youthful behave in a very similar fashion, but for the young chicken, the puppy, and the young chimpanzee life has much to teach which is learned with great readiness.

Instinct and Intelligence. This distinction between instinct and intelligence is sometimes difficult to grasp, largely because ' intelligence ' is an ambiguous word. As opposed to ' instinct ' it means only that the behaviour which shows it is due in part to the *individual* past history, the *acquired* experience of the animal. Intelligent behaviour, in other words, depends upon *retention*, and retention we studied in the last chapter. Instinctive behaviour, by contrast, is due to innate congenital factors. All behaviour, even that of the genius among men, is a blend of the two, though the relative importance of *congenital* and *acquired* factors varies enormously. But there is another sense of ' intelligence ' which confuses this distinction. The fatuous performance of a ' blue-bottle ' on a window-pane provides a good example. Relevant circumstances have changed, but the fly's behaviour remains the same. Hence we tend to judge the ' intelligence ' of a performance by its appropriateness. But we should remember that some purely instinctive conduct is extraordinarily apt, and that intelligence can lead to disastrous follies.

The essential distinction lies in the extent to which congenital and acquired factors are governing the behaviour.

The Process of Learning. Almost all behaviour, we have said, is a blend of the two. How exactly do these two factors co-operate? And are we right in regarding them as separate factors? Let us consider a simple case. A newly hatched chick begins very early to peck at and swallow small objects. This is instinctive behaviour. At first it may get one in five of the objects pecked at; after ten days it gets four out of five, which seems to be the best it can do. The improvement is partly due to learning and partly to maturation. As it grows older its instinctive arrangements work better, but exercise assists this maturation. So far as learning is at work, intelligence, in its lowliest form, is showing itself. The same thing happens with the flight of even the young. It improves. But before long the chicken pecks at something, orange peel, for example, which is distasteful. The peel is at once rejected. Now note what occurs after a few of these distressing experiences. In the normal case, even though hungry, it refrains entirely from pecking. Something has been

acquired which modifies its behaviour. The
sight of the peel no longer prompts the
natural instinctive response. What exactly
has happened? This process, known as
' acquirement of meaning ', is so important
and psychologists are so at variance upon
the account to be given, that a close study
is very desirable. It leads us straight to
the central principle involved in the growth
of the mind.

The Modification of Responses. On
the first occasion congenital arrangements
in the chicken's brain cause it first to peck
at and then to reject the peel. Thus the
pecking-seizing-swallowing sequence is upset.
And the co-ordination centre which responded
to the situation by setting this sequence in
action is left just as in the case of Pavlov's
dog, in a new state of tuning due to the
backwash influence of the rejection-response
or of the taste. This new state of tuning
disconnects the peel situation from its former
response. Next time the peel is spied the
centre is not discharged. The chicken passes
the peel by. And its behaviour is entirely
explained by the working of retention ; what
is retained being not the former set of
responses nor the former experience but a new

tuning, a new modification of the disposition.

In order that past experience shall assist in controlling present behaviour with a view (as it appears) to the future, it is not in the least necessary that it should be revived in the form of memory. The chick need not *remember* that the peel tasted unpleasant. It need not, in fact, be conscious at all, though there are fairly good reasons based on general analogies for supposing that it has some kind of simple consciousness. Probably the peel simply looks unattractive to it. Such arguments as are valid on this point largely depend on analogy from our own experience. When we refuse a dish we commonly feel just disinclined to partake of it ; we do not, as a rule, remember former occasions on which it disagreed with us. Some people do, but only as a result of giving a kind of attention to their food which it is very unlikely that the chick can give. When by a judicious wriggle we avoid falling off a bicycle we do not need to remember former falls. As we shall see later, far more of our behaviour is ordinarily governed by such *unconscious* action of the traces of the past than by conscious recollection, revival, deliberation, and decision.

This temptation to suppose that the only way in which we can learn by experience is by remembering it, and by bringing our memories to bear upon the present circumstances, is responsible for most of the trouble which the theory of instinct has caused the psychologist. At present it is causing great difficulties to psycho-analysis. If we realize from the outset that incidents of our past constantly and continuously affect our present behaviour without our having any consciousness of them, we shall be spared much bewilderment when we come to consider what *the unconscious* may be and how to conceive it. We shall avoid also attributing too much consciousness to animals, and in particular endowing them with conscious prevision or foresight of the ends which they seek and achieve. We are much less conscious and less prescient ourselves than we suppose.

Intelligence and instinct are not, we have seen, rival or opposed forces. Intelligence is the means by which, through experience, we refine and elaborate the play of the instincts.

Trial and Error. Now that the not very interesting chicken has served its purpose, we can pass to more elaborate forms of animal behaviour, in experiments on trial and error. Let us consider that ingenious contraption, the puzzle-box. A cat with a need for fish is placed in a box from which it can only escape to gain access to the fish by pulling a string. The times taken on a number of successive attempts are recorded. It is found that they tend to grow less and less. The number of random movements which the cat makes decreases, not smoothly, but as a general tendency. Finally the cat learns to make the required kind of movement immediately. Often this learning takes place with remarkable suddenness. Now suppose that after the cat has learned to pull the string at once when it is hanging as a loop in one corner of the cage, we arrange the loop to hang in the middle of the box. What does the cat do? A bright cat is not found to repeat the whole series of random scratchings and clawings which originally led to its learning how to escape. Instead, after perhaps a claw or two at the place where the loop used to hang, it finds the loop in its new position and pulls it at once. This shows that it has 'grasped the connection', as we are tempted to say, between pulling the loop and escape. The problem is to

discover what this 'grasping of the connection' consists in. Is it a matter of
'insight' by the cat, or can it be accounted
for merely by the stamping in of acquired
responses?

It is important to realize how difficult the
problem really is, and the best way to do this
is to consider some of the theories which
have been put forward and how far they
succeed or fail as explanations.

The accepted view of learning held until
recently by most experimenters in animal
psychology (Thorndike has been the initiator
of most of these investigations) was in broad
outline this. Three laws were supposed to
co-operate : the Law of Effect, the Law of
Recency, the Law of Exercise. Different
authorities have stressed these laws in different degrees. We are already familiar with
them all. The Law of Effect is that, other
things being equal, success leads to the
repetition of a response, failure to its elimina-
tion. The Law of Recency is that, other
things being equal, the last response is the
one which has the best chance of recurring.
The Law of Exercise is simply that repetition
of any response tends to confirm it. By these
three laws the response actually retained was

supposed to be picked out of an original infinitely varied range of possible random instinctive responses, all equally likely to be made.

The selection was supposed to be a ' blind ' selection, not guided by any observation. " The cat learns to get out by getting out, not by seeing how to get out ", is Woodworth's summary of this view.

One difficulty will probably have occurred to the reader. The theory might work if the movement finally made by the cat was always *exactly* the same. But in actual fact it is a certain *kind* of movement, not a perfectly specific movement, which is in the end adopted. The objection gets still more force when we find that the cat *transfers* the learned response to a different situation, pulling the loop at a different level and from a new angle. Quite different movements may then be required, prompted by quite different views of the loop. So that we cannot be content with any theory which deals with this kind of learning purely in terms of movements and stimuli. For the movements and stimuli are never exactly repeated. Learning, therefore, cannot be an establishment of firm connections between particular stimuli and particular movements. None the less, as a reaction to the older, anthropomorphic views which supposed the cat to reason the matter out, to act, in fact, just as we should if we were remarkably stupid, this theory was a great advance in the right direction.

Perception in Cats. We are forced back, then, to the question, What is a response ? What is it that is learned ? And to answer this we must take stock anew of the whole situation. There is the cat boxed up, consumed by a lust for fish ; and generally in an unsettled condition. Its whole activity must be regarded as the elaborate way in which this disturbance settles down. In some way plainly the actual experience of the cat when it finally pulls the loop, the particular state it is in at that moment, is the thing which matters.

We are here concerned with the working of the co-ordination centres discussed in our account of the brain, and the number of repetitions required to fix a new type of pattern for the cat. What is acquired is not a particular response, but a disposition, just as we saw must be the case with the chicken and the peel ; in this case a disposition to perceive the loop as 'something to be pulled' and as the beginning of a transition towards escape. The cat's world does now contain a new kind of thing. Its receptive centres are capable of handling a new pattern—and this, but nothing more than this, is what is meant by insight.

CHAPTER VII

THE MENTALITY OF APES

Köhler's Apes. We can now pass to the study of the animals which are the nearest relatives of man, and it is to Wolfgang Köhler that we are indebted for a study of the mind of the chimpanzee which is already a landmark in the history of animal psychology.

The great advantage of Köhler's experiments is that they set problems which, if insight or understanding occurs in apes, they might be expected to solve by this means—by the formation, that is to say, of new configurations, new dispositions or *Gestalts*.[1] The cat could not well be expected to master the mechanical construction of its box, since essential parts of it were quite

[1] Professor Köhler of Berlin, in *The Mentality of Apes* (3rd Edition, 1931), has given a full account of his experiments in Tenerife, and both he and Professor Koffka, in *The Growth of the Mind* (5th Edition, 1931), have used the word *Gestalt* to refer to a disposition, conceived not as a fixed pathway among neurones, but as a system with an end-state to which it tends to return when disturbed.

hidden. But Köhler's apes, being given much simpler tasks, had an opportunity of really showing what they could do.

We will take what was perhaps the cleverest performance of Sultan, the most intelligent of Köhler's apes. Apes vary in intelligence almost as much as men do. All the animals easily mastered the use of sticks in dragging fruit placed outside the cage within reach. And from the very start they would place the stick correctly behind the fruit in order to draw it forward. There were no random movements. If the stick to be used lay so that both stick and fruit were visible together, there was, as a rule, no delay, but if they were widely separated, difficulties arose at first. The stick did not easily enter into the situation. It remained indifferent to the animal, 'something to bite upon' or 'something to jump with' or 'to throw', not 'something to fetch fruit with'. In other words, the stick has to be perceived in a special way before it can be used ; it has to be seen as a tool, as a step or link in the transition by which the end-state of securing the fruit is gained.

The Construction of Tools. The elaborate experiments of Nadie Kohts in Moscow

(1914-16) were chiefly devoted to showing that vision plays a predominant rôle in the perceptions of the chimpanzee, and Köhler's observations are particularly interesting on this point. Two sticks are often put together so that they *look* like one long stick, and the ape will then try to use them as such, regardless of the fact that they do not stay together and are *practically* useless. But can two jointed sticks be combined so as to become technically useful? Sultan was the first to solve the problem. For more than an hour he failed, poking about in various ways, but although he several times put one stick exactly to the opening of the other he made no attempt to fit them together. Even a suggestion from the observer who put one finger into the opening of the stick under the animal's nose (without pointing to the other stick at all) was of no assistance.

A little later, when sitting with his back to the fruit, Sultan happened to find himself holding one rod in either hand so that they were in a straight line ; he pushed the thinner one a little way into the opening of the thicker, jumped up, ran immediately towards the railings, and began to draw a banana towards him with the double stick. Though the sticks fell apart, Sultan at once replaced them, and proceeded with the greatest assurance to rake fruit towards him, replacing the sticks whenever they slipped asunder. The proceeding so pleased him that without stopping to eat any of the fruit, he continued to rake into his cage everything that he could reach. The contrast of this mode of discovery with the supposed . blind random scratchings of the cat in the puzzle-box is very striking.

Building Experiments. The building performances of the apes are especially interesting because of the resemblance they show to the young child's performances with his bricks. Bananas would be hung up so that the ape had to pile one box upon another to reach them. Dragging a box to the right place and standing on it for a leap was easily learned. So even was the placing in some fashion of another box on top of it. The same suddenness of the discovery was noticed here as in the case of the double stick. Sultan when he failed would seize a box and gallop all round the room with it, showing every sign of annoyance; not in order to use the box in building, but to give vent to his temper. This suggests that a good many of the cat's supposed random movements in the puzzle-box may have really nothing to do with escape, but be merely the cat's way of resenting the situation.

The ape's chief difficulty in building is not to see that one box can be put upon another ; it is to see how to put it so that it will stay there. And this difficulty the chimpanzee apparently cannot completely solve any more than the child at a certain stage in its play with bricks can solve it. The chimpanzee has practically no statics. He will poise one box corner-wise upon another, trying meanwhile " with concentrated gravity to ascend the pinnacle. With an amazing stubbornness and minute care, one of the apes, Grande, repeated this masterly mistake for years ". Often her extraordinary gifts as an equilibrist lead to triumph. Grande in the photograph (Plate I) is retaining her painfully constructed edifice in equilibrium only through a careful distribution of her own weight. Unfortunately everything depends upon her not letting go of the bananas or pulling them down. A catastrophe occurred immediately after the photograph was taken. The other ape is the genius Sultan, who has been forbidden

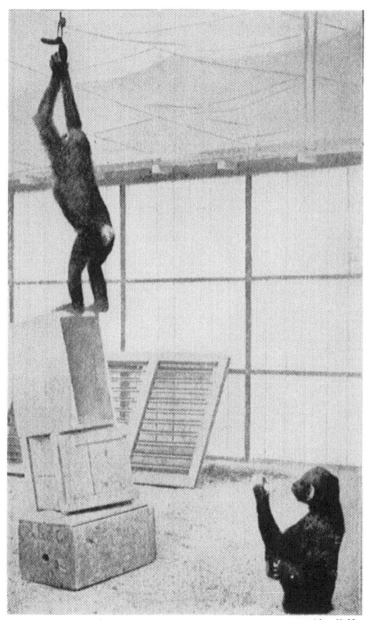

PLATE I

to take part in the building ; the sympathetic participation shown in his left hand should be especially noticed.

Needs and Instincts. So far we have paid attention chiefly to the development of intelligence ; this of course is only one aspect of the animal's mental growth, though it is the aspect which has been most studied. We have seen, however, that the animal's intelligent acts are all prompted by some definite need or set of needs, though we have kept somewhat monotonously to manifestations of one need only, the need for food. The reason is that this is the motive most convenient to the experimenter. But the animal's needs are various and the question naturally arises, How do the chimpanzee's needs compare with those of man, and what light do his presumably simpler needs throw upon our own, upon our desires, and the working of our passions in general?

We must distinguish between the animal's innate needs and its acquired needs. Most of man's needs and many of those of the higher animals, especially the domesticated animals, are acquired ; they are, as it were, grafted on primitive needs in the manner described in Chapter V. The chimpanzee needs no boxes or fishing rods in its wild condition, and if we consider only congenital needs our question plainly is the one which has been so often asked, namely, How many instincts are there ?   To this, different answers have been given corresponding to the psychologist's purpose in raising the question.   Thus Freud, having in view as simple and fundamental a classification of human instincts as possible, classifies them into two groups, ego-instincts and sex-instincts ;   while Thorndike, wishing to keep close to the facts, is content to list an indefinite number of specific situations with the instinctive responses which they elicit.

The Classification of Instincts.   Another kind of answer is McDougall's, based definitely upon a theory of the relation of instinct to emotion.   Emotion for McDougall is "a mode of experience which accompanies the working within us of instinctive impulses ", and each instinct, "no matter how brought into play, is accompanied by its own peculiar quality of experience which may be called a primary emotion."

McDougall's list of instincts is as follows :

Instincts	*Emotional Qualities*
1. Instinct of escape (of self-preservation, of avoidance, danger instinct).	Fear (terror, fright, alarm, trepidation).

Instincts	*Emotional Qualities*
2. Instinct of combat (aggression, pugnacity).	Anger (rage, fury, annoyance, irritation, displeasure).
3. Repulsion (repugnance).	Disgust (nausea, loathing, repugnance).
4. Parental (protective).	Tender emotion (love, tenderness, tender feeling).
5. Appeal.	Distress (feeling of helplessness).
6. Pairing (mating, reproduction, sexual).	Lust (sexual emotion or excitement, sometimes called love).
7. Curiosity (inquiry, discovery, investigation).	Curiosity (feeling of mystery, of strangeness, of wonder).
8. Submission (self-abasement).	Feeling of subjection (of inferiority, devotion, etc.).
9. Assertion (self-display).	Elation (feeling of superiority, masterfulness, pride).
10. Social or gregarious instinct.	Feeling of loneliness, of isolation, nostalgia.
11. Food-seeking (hunting).	Appetite or craving in narrower sense (gusto).
12. Acquisition (hoarding instinct).	Feeling of ownership, of possession (protectivity).
13. Construction.	Feeling of creativeness, of making, of productivity.
14. Laughter.	Amusement (jollity, carelessness, relaxation).

Besides the emotions here mentioned McDougall also recognizes blended and secondary emotions (such as horror, awe, gratitude, and scorn) and derived emotions (such as joy, sorrow, surprise, anxiety, hope, and despair). The last spring from the facilitation or obstruction of desires. But even with the addition of such further complexities it is difficult to see why the particular emotional qualities in the list should be chosen rather than these, as the accompaniment of the instinct. Each of McDougall's instincts seems to have not a single primary emotion attached to it, but a cycle of distinctive emotions.

A More Fundamental Division. For the purposes of scientific anthropology something more fundamental is clearly required ; and a classification based on the primary and derivative needs discussed in Chapter V will provide the essentials. Thus pairing and food-seeking, together with what McDougall describes as the ' minor instincts ' of urination and defecation, occur cyclically as a result of internal needs—like sleeping and waking, and organic processes such as breathing and digestion ;   whereas escape, combat (except perhaps in Irishmen), and repugnance only occur in connection with fairly specific external situations.   In other words, instinctive responses of internal origin correspond to the primitive organic needs which we have been discussing above.   These can legitimately be called drives, while the others are of the nature of readjustments arising through the obstruction or complication of such prior activities.   Such an

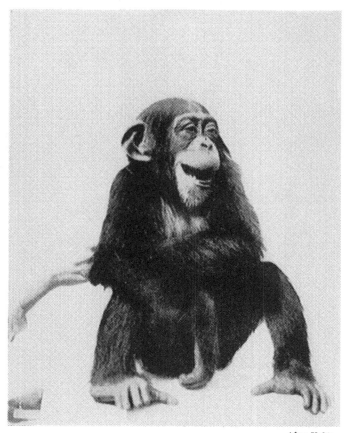

PLATE II. CHIMPANZEE LAUGHING
(or not ?)

adjustment repeated frequently enough may become a derivative drive. Thus escape is a development of the much more primitive impulse to remove the skin from stimuli which threaten to destroy tissue ; and flight from a loud noise is to be explained in terms of pre-human conditioning. The social instincts arise partly from sex and partly from the need to co-operate in hunting or housing problems.

The Value of McDougall's Scheme. Apart from theoretical considerations, McDougall's scheme, being in accord with popular language, gives us a rough-and-ready means of comparing different animal species in their responses to similar general situations, and of comparing the behaviour of the animal in varying situations. If the reader will try to analyse the behaviour of his dog, or that of his friends, by asking which of these instincts on various occasions are primarily concerned, he will soon discover that the list is very serviceable. As a problem picture we include a photograph of a chimpanzee which seems to have a more direct bearing on the still disputed occurrence of genuine amusement in an animal than any hitherto published.

The Dangers of Anthropomorphism.
In all these inquiries we must be chary of
lending the animal, when it behaves much
as we might do, mental processes similar in
all respects to our own. Some apparently
highly altruistic animal behaviour, for example, is, when closely examined, found to
be very much simpler in its motives. The
broody hen sits on her eggs not through
any passion of maternal love, but to allay a
local inflammation ; and a capon suitably
irritated with pepper can be turned into a
most devoted foster-mother. Kirkman, with
the black-headed gull, found that the bird
does not resent the removal of her eggs, and
would sit for the full incubating period on
any object that is not too uncomfortable,
such as a small square or circular box, or a
golf-ball.[1]

Our own emotions are the clue to any
scheme of instincts in so far as they allow us
to classify our main activities, and the main
kinds of situations which call them forth.
We then look for similar activities and situations in animal behaviour. But we do not,
or should not, suppose that the emotions

[1] To appear in his forthcoming *The Expression of Emotion
in Birds*.

After Kohts

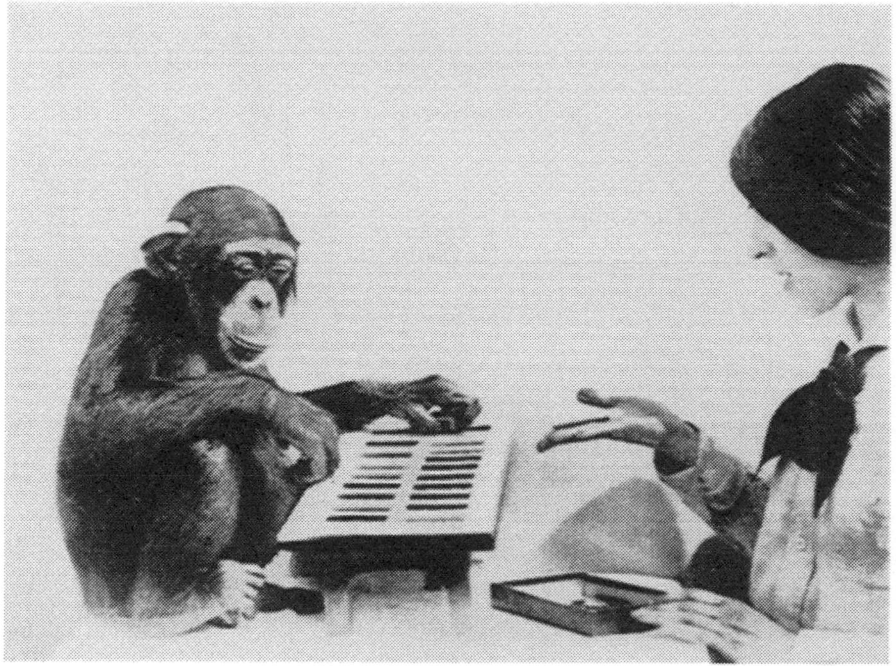

PLATE III. CHIMPANZEE MATCHING COLOURS

of animals very different in development from ourselves need have much in common with our own.

With this very necessary precaution in mind we can briefly consider some of the main features of animal behaviour which are significant for human psychology.

Naturally the nearer we come to man in the biological tree the more significant is the behaviour. The passions of the ant, of the cuttlefish, or of the crocodile, could we divine them, would tell us little about our own ; but with the chimpanzee the case is altogether different. We can both conjecture them with some probability and draw comparisons with profit ; but the experiments of Nadie Kohts, to which reference has already been made, and one of which is illustrated in Plate III, suggest that more depends on the skill and understanding of the human observer than has usually been supposed.

The Social Life of Apes. Group phenomena are among the most interesting in this respect, for the chimpanzee's strongest and most varied emotions arise through his membership of a group.[1] As Professor

[1] In his *Social Life in the Animal World* (1927) Professor Alverdes has surveyed the whole field of animal psychology in its social aspects.

Köhler points out, " A chimpanzee kept in solitude is not a real chimpanzee at all." An ape separated from his fellows will risk his very life to get back to them. The group, however, shows less interest in the separated one. He will stretch his arms imploringly towards them, howling and whimpering, and if they do not come to comfort him, will wave sticks towards them, and even throw things towards them, not out of anger, but in order to do something, no matter what, in their direction as a relief to his feelings. This tendency to do something in the direction of whatever is the object of the emotion is very general. And what is done is not necessarily at all useful.

The return of the lost one is the occasion for general rejoicings. The whole group becomes very lively ; they put their arms round him, " even beat him a little for pleasure ". An attack upon one member of the group often produces an extraordinary disturbance. The whole group sets up a howl, as if with one voice. It seems certain that one chimpanzee will genuinely defend another, and not in his own interest. But they differ amazingly in this respect as in other points of character. Thus some chimpanzees rarely incite the others to mass-attack, but the gifted Sultan, always inclined to pose as a martyr, continually did so. He seems, in fact, to have borne a remarkable resemblance to many human geniuses; for instance, in his dislike of uninteresting jobs.

The actual sight of suffering will prompt behaviour which looks in the highest degree solicitous and maternal, but with chimpanzees ' out of sight is out of mind '. *The ape seems to have practically no power of imagining.* Expressions of emotion which have no connection with the animal's material advantage are common. When punished, an imperious desire for forgiveness may be shown; the animal will make up to his humàn companion with apish protests of friendship. Chimpanzees ·instantly take to little children and infants.

The study of the sexual life of chimpanzees is of particular interest.[1] It clearly has a bearing upon the vexed question of the Freudian theory of infantile sexuality. " It seems to me," writes Köhler, " that among these creatures sexual excitement is less

[1] See S. Zuckerman, *The Social Life of Monkeys and Apes,* 1931.

specific and less differentiated from any other kind of excitement than among human beings. We may almost say that any strong emotion, and thus any strong external stimulus, tends to react directly upon both the colon and the genitals, but not so as to give the impression of exaggerated and concentrated sexuality, but rather of an inner vehemence and interdependence of all vivid inner processes."

Terror and Curiosity. When in doubt chimpanzees scratch their heads. When surprised or apprehensive or startled they display entirely human gestures. When frightened they fly or cling together ; it is an intriguing fact that they were most terrified by certain small stuffed toys, cloth donkeys with black buttons for eyes. It is tempting to connect this peculiar terror with the influence which effigies so mysteriously exert in the lives of primitive people.

Finally, for we must pass on to study these same activities in the child and in man, the chimpanzees recognized objects in photographs and, having been introduced to mirrors, thenceforward would spend hours studying reflections of themselves and of other things in pools, bright pieces of tin, and tiny splinters of glass. " What strange beings ", as Köhler remarks, " to be permanently attracted by the contemplation of such phenomena, which can bring them not the least tangible or ' practical ' benefit ! "

H

CHAPTER VIII

MENTAL GROWTH IN MAN

THAT apish cousin of the chimpanzee from whom we descend probably differed from him in two important respects as well as in matters of degree. One was that he developed free images, and the other that he took to using speech.

The Development and Uses of Imagery. The power to form images corresponding to the things we have perceived is one of the most mysterious, as it is one of the most obvious, of our talents. It is an entirely open question whether images may not occur in the mental processes of even lowly animals.

But the child, by the time he reaches the story-telling age (about four), beyond all doubt makes extensive use of images, and in two fashions. He uses them for practical purposes, in solving problems, and he uses them for emotional gratification, in fantasy or daydreaming, as part of the absorbing activity of play.

An image (see Chapter III) is essentially a perception taking place without the normal stimulation, without the incoming impulses from the sense-organs which perception demands. It is usual to divide images up into types—visual, auditory, kinæsthetic, etc. —corresponding to the sense-organs which would have to be stimulated for the corresponding perceptions. But this classification is somewhat artificial. We shall see later (Chapter XII) that most perceptions are very complicated, including commonly a variety of sensory factors. We perceive a table not only with our eyes, but through the effects of past handlings of it, for example. Correspondingly, an image of a table is rarely a purely visual affair, but more complicated. Sometimes, of course, one aspect will be more prominent than another. A few individuals appear to be entirely without imagery. For most people their power of imaging varies with their physiological state, being notably increased with the onset of sleep. Those much engaged in abstract thought are believed to have their normal imaging-power impaired. These differences sometimes make psychology unduly mysterious to beginners who happen to differ in their natural imagery from the authors they read. On the other hand, since a man's imagery is the part or aspect of his mind which he himself can most easily investigate, images have tended to take too prominent a position in psychology ever since the time of Locke, whose 'way of ideas' made images the foundation-stone of the theory of the mind.

In the child the first appearance of the images is difficult to trace, just as in the ape. There is, further, reason to think that the distinction between actual perceiving and imaging is not, at an early age, nearly so clear cut as it is in adults. This sharp separation of the actual from the imaged is one of the many differences between the adult's world and the child's. It is maintained by investigators of 'eidetics' (Gk. 'eidos' = image) that the majority of children under fourteen project their images into the external world, and that many adults never get beyond this infantile stage. In Chapter XIV the importance of other forms of projection will also be considered.

Extensive use of imagery in practical affairs seems likely to be a development subsequent to this use of it as a direct though bodiless and illusory satisfier of needs. For wide experience and a very considerable plasticity are necessary before imagery becomes of real practical service. We commonly think of our imagery as guiding our action. We imagine what we are going to do, and then do it, so runs the traditional account. But ninety-nine times out of a hundred—as anyone who watches himself at all closely will agree—we actually do something else when the moment comes. Circumstances must govern our perceptions and guide us to the satisfaction of our needs ; our preliminary imaginings, prompted by our needs alone, cannot. Imagining, in fact, if it gets out of hand is a great danger. An enormous number of the catastrophes of the mind can be traced to just this, to phantasy which is blocking the ways of perception and substituting an illusory satisfaction for an actual solution of the problem.

But if images are not as directly useful as we often suppose, imagining, none the less, has an indirect value as an exercise of our powers of perception. Through much imagining (if not too stereotyped) the mind may become more plastic, more able to form new perceptions, when the occasion demands it.

Play. Memory begins in a rudimentary form early in the second year, but remains very indefinite for a long while. " Even for a four-year-old child a definite remembrance of yesterday is difficult, and one of the day before impossible. At this age there exists a vague impression of happenings long past, likewise a rough distinction between before and after, and occasionally one between to-day and not to-day." [1]

This vagueness and indeterminateness of memory in the child is probably connected with the predominance of play in its life. We shall never understand play—the most extensive activity of the most important period of our lives—either in general or in its particularities, unless we realize that the child's world is almost entirely unlike ours. All his perceptions differ from ours, not only in definiteness, but in kind. The description and analysis of this difference is a very valuable achievement of modern

---

[1] K. Koffka, *The Growth of the Mind*, p. 244. This may be the reason why we find it difficult to recall infantile experiences. Another reason is repression (cf. Chapter XIII). A third may be the slight extent to which a child verbalizes his experiences (cf. Watson, *Behaviorism* (1925), p. 209), and a fourth is probably to be found in the fact that, since the child's world is so unlike ours, memories of it would be of little use to us, and would involve repression (cf. Chapter XV). When we have mastered a subject it is peculiarly difficult to recall our first crude conceptions of it.

psychology, not only because an unsympathetic failure to realize it on the part of parents and others is bad for the child, but also because the common alternative, sentimental nonsense about it, is even worse.

The child's world differs from the adult's because his interests are different. The majority of the adult's interests do not yet exist for him, and therefore the ways of perceiving which are going later to serve those interests do not exist either. Pre-eminently that way of perceiving things which springs from the endeavour to see them as they are does not yet exist. It is true that adults differ among themselves in this respect, but their differences, however important, are slight if we compare them with the child. The young child perceives things *only* in their relation to his own needs and desires, and his world is a reflection of his own inner activities.

To understand what this implies we must consider the peculiar, the unique helplessness of the infant. The young guinea-pig is independent of its mother in three days' time, the young white rat in thirty; the young human being is still very dependent after three thousand days. This long subordination is, as has often been remarked, the secret of man's superiority, but it is also the clue to much which is less satisfactory in him. As we shall see, it has consequences which he must eliminate when he finally grows up, as well as consequences which he must retain.

Infantile Perception. The helpless dependence of the infant upon those who tend him affects his perceptions from the beginning. His first differentiated reactions to sounds are aroused by the human voice. He takes an interest in faces as early as his twenty-fifth day ; even in the second month of his life the face and voice of his mother may cause him to laugh. After three months the recognition has developed in differentiation, and thereafter the child behaves quite differently towards familiar persons and to strangers. Facial expressions influence him by the time he is six months old. But what *we* should regard as simple forms are not distinguished until much later. The letter O, for example, not till the end of a year. These, if we consider them, are very remarkable facts. They imply that the infant is building up a view of the world very unlike that which at first sight we should suppose

it to be forming. Unless we are careful
we tend to think that the infant's world
begins for him as a multitudinous chaos of
lights and contacts and noises, " a big buzz-
ing blooming confusion ", as James put it,
out of which he collects elements together
and gradually combines them into groups
which become for him separate things. His
mother's face on this view would be a
combination of countless sensations, and its
various expressions indescribably complex
distributions of light and shade. But in
fact nothing of the kind is going on. The
infant does not proceed from the simple to
the complex ; he begins with what bio-
logically matters for him, and this in nearly
all cases is complex.

Thus the infant's early outfit consists of
perceptions, not perceptions of colours, spots,
sounds, and touches as such, but of expressions
of patterns which favour or thwart his
activities ; and on this basis of perceptions
he continues to build up his world, for it
is a fundamental law of the mind that so
long as it can it will use perceptions already
acquired rather than form new ones. The
child who calls a badger the first time it sees
one a ' bow-wow ' and the philosopher who

tries to bring new facts under his old headings are obvious instances. Conversely, the child's comparatively undeveloped power of recognition and discrimination are due to its lack of experience of the ways in which signs change from situation to situation.

Primitive Mentality. The world of the child continues for a long while to be modelled for him on these patterns ; and is therefore informed with intention towards him. Not that he explicitly supposes it to be alive or to be thinking and willing about him. To do this would imply that he made a distinction between the conscious and the unconscious, which in fact he cannot yet make. He simply has only one way of regarding it. In this respect his world resembles that of primitive man, and the comparison between the child's mind and that of certain people of rude culture is illuminating.

All over the world, in Australia, in Africa, in Melanesia, and in the Arctic Circle, are to be found peoples for whom the idea of a mere accident in serious affairs even in the most obvious cases does not arise. When a man falls from a tree through trusting to a rotten branch, or when he is snapped up by a crocodile, or dies of a snake bite, or has his head cut open in battle, the view taken is that some enemy, not his own carelessness, or the branch, the crocodile, the snake, or even necessarily the opposing swordsman, is ultimately responsible. Even his death through old age is put down to sorcery, and this view is arrived at not, as we might suppose, through elaborate and muddled ratiocination based upon a few misleading instances, but simply because the idea of an important happening undirected by some intention is too difficult for them to form. Their only way of perceiving serious events is to regard them as caused by some intention. Thus, a sorcerer by his magic must have made the man fall, or entered into the crocodile or the snake, or deprived the warrior of his accustomed skill in guarding his head. The primitive thinker, in fact, will only ask questions which begin with 'why'.[1] Mere matters of 'how' seem to him trivial. He will point out that the crocodile snapped up one man rather than another, or snapped him up to-day, but not yesterday, and he

[1] Cf. J. Piaget, *Language and Thought of the Child*, 1926, for a masterly analysis of the questions asked by a child of seven. The continuation of Piaget's studies, *Judgment and Reasoning in the Child* (1928) has been followed by a translation of his three subsequent volumes, on Representation, Cause, and Moral Judgment.

is not content with any explanation which does not reduce this to somebody's intention ; so he continues to bathe just as before in crocodile-infested waters, confident that the saurians will not harm him unless charged thereto by the malice of some sorcerer.

What he regards as the practical step is to seek out and slaughter the sorcerer ; for a mere slaughter of crocodiles would only lead to his choosing some other means whereby to wreak his malice. This behaviour will seem to us unbelievably obtuse unless we realize the mental peculiarity in which it is rooted. It is a consequence of the primitive's way of perceiving events ; his set of perceptions takes no account of events which are not directed at somebody by somebody else. But to understand how this way of perceiving accidents comes to be so preposterously fixed, we have to notice another characteristic of primitive mentality, namely the prodigious influence of society upon it. In any group in which no difference of opinion exists it is almost impossible for an individual to dissent from the common doctrine. We shall shortly have to consider again this influence of society, of the common doctrine and the common practice, on the individual mind. Even in the most highly civilized communities it is still overwhelmingly powerful. But our present task is to describe the world of the child.

The Play World and the Real World. His world, we have said, is the reflection of his interests, and since these interests are simpler than the adult's, his is a different world. But besides being simpler they are more separate. For the adult and in the degree to which he differs from a child, nearly all his activities are linked together and mutually influence one another. What he does in the morning is influenced by what he is going to do in the afternoon and so on. In other words, his various interests are integrated, though never perfectly. In the child this integration has hardly begun. And this probably explains the tardy development of systematic memory in him. His life is a multitude of pieces rather than a fabric, and his world corresponds. Thus a shift of interest has an effect upon his world which to the adult is difficult to comprehend. The block which ten minutes ago was an automobile suddenly becomes something to throw about, and the next moment may turn into a tree. How are we to picture these changes in the child's way of perceiving it ?

In the first place we must be clear that there is no question of any actual illusion. If the block could be actually turned by magic into a tree or an automobile, the child would be as surprised as we should. On the other hand, his perceptions of it are certainly more plastic than ours, because they are less definite, and so at the same time are his perceptions of a tree and of an automobile. We regard the block consistently as a wooden cube, but to the child it is only something which favours now one and now another of his interests. We can, if we like, get him to see it as we see it, but only by giving him an interest in so doing. We can use his desire to please us or be flattered by us, for example. Similarly with trees and automobiles. They are not to him the intricate objects which they are to us, but only things which excite him in different ways, and these excitements are still easily detachable from their objects. For in us a block and an automobile are each inextricably fixed in extensive and conflicting systems of interests. But the child's interests do not yet ramify and are still fluid. We get nearest to his condition sometimes in our dreams when we treat one thing as though it was another without any difficulty or doubt, but at the same time without any illusion.

This plasticity of the child's world is gradually broken into by the demands which adults make upon him. A certain number of his activities are allowed free course, others are controlled ; so a separation grows up between the world of adults and his own world. The adult's world hangs together and has a consistency from which his own world is free. But it is, therefore, a world full of opposition, constantly denying possibilities which his own world can realize. Thus a struggle may arise between the two worlds, the world of reality, as we may call it, and the world of desire or make-believe ; and the outcome of this struggle is often decisive for the individual's character and personality.

The Conflict with Reality. The two worlds interact curiously. Little by little the distinctions and interconnections forced on the child by the actual world get taken over into his play world. And as the division between them grows clearer to him, the attractions of the play world increase. In the play world he is master ; in the other world of the adult he is constantly being coerced. But as more and more of the consistent patterns of the actual world get taken over into play, freedom here becomes more difficult. The crisis comes when the play world through this limitation—through the degree in which it has taken over patterns from the actual world—begins to offer difficulties to the child. Two paths are open to him. He may break up these patterns again and so lapse back into a freer, more ' unreal ' kind of activity, or he may be driven by these difficulties in the direction of an increased mastery of the actual world. The compromises which result from these difficult adjustments will occupy us later in Chapter XV.

To speak of this as a crisis is perhaps misleading ; it is not a single event ; it is a struggle which always lasts many years and may last a whole lifetime, and it arises not over one difficulty, but at innumerable points. It may be decided in one way for some clashes, and in the opposite way for others. To take a typical example : though schoolmasters for good and obvious reasons encourage the confusion, play and games are really entirely different activities. Most people can remember something of the process of transition, and perhaps, too, something of the resentment the child feels when the grown-up first attempts this particular interference with his play. An afternoon spent with a bat and a ball, and perhaps one or two friends (though these are not strictly necessary) who really participate in the activity, every stroke being a performance only to be equalled by a Perry or a Bradman, is one thing. A tense and humiliating endeavour to rival the *actual* performances of older and more skilled companions, or to escape their derision, is quite another. It is not play at all, but actual life in one of its most searching forms. Games, in fact, are one of the chief instruments by which the play world is broken down.

The result of this and innumerable similar conflicts is a certain balance between the amount and kind of energy which the individual devotes to actual affairs (including games) and the amount and kind devoted to genuine play which little by little becomes fantasy or daydreaming. Most people have one or two lines, often unknown to anyone, along which they continue all their lives to play—that is, to dream, not to act ; offshoots as it were of the original dream-world which have never been drawn into the larger unity of coherent waking purposes. These are a common cause of mental troubles ; for, as we shall see, they lead to the setting up of unreal standards, of ideals which can never be attained in the actual world. The dreamer remains in a state of constant dissatisfaction with any substitute offered for his dream-image, or unconsciously takes refuge in illness to evade the test of public achievement.

CHAPTER IX

MAN'S LINGUISTIC HERITAGE

Speech. The chief social influences exerted on the child come about through *speech*. The importance of speech in human psychology is even yet generally underestimated. It is not too much to say that our minds differ from those of the animals because of speech. Its discovery was probably the origin of man.[1]

Expressions and Names. Even in the chimpanzee, as we have seen, and in many far lower animals, a rudimentary form of speech is found. The dog barks and whines, the frog croaks, and. the cat's virtuosity is well known, but it is better to give these prehuman manifestations of vocal powers

[1] G. Elliot Smith, " The Evolution of Intelligence," in *Problems of Personality, Studies in Honour of Dr. Morton Prince*, pp. 6-7. A very original account of everything that modern phonetics and the study of tongue ' gestures ' can contribute to our understanding both of the past and the future of vocal utterance will be found in Sir Richard Paget's *Human Speech* (1929), where what may be called a ' Tongue-young ' theory is added to the standard ' bow-wow ', ' ding-dong ', ' pooh-pooh', and other explanations of linguistic origins.

another name. We must regard them as *expressions* of the animal's activities ; in most cases they will be expressions of fairly well marked emotions, and this merely expressive use of sounds must be clearly distinguished from their use in *naming*, though of course many sounds have both functions.

The difference, though simple, is very fundamental. A merely expressive cry arises directly from the animal's need, his want, his desire, his joy or fear, his interest in general, and *it varies with this activity*. But a naming cry arises from the perception of a given state of affairs and *varies with this state of affairs*. Briefly we express ourselves alike because *we* are alike ; we name things alike because *they* are alike. Plainly naming cannot arise until the animal can respond to situations not merely as eliciting this or that activity but as possessing this or that character. Naming itself is of course an expression of a need, and all use of speech involves expression ; but some vocal activity also involves what is known technically as *objective reference*, and it is this further use of speech which is man's peculiar achievement.

It will help us to imagine some of the

steps in this distinctively human ' misuse
of language '[1] if we realize how confused
(from our adult point of view) both the
animal and the infant are. We make a
distinction between our emotions, which are
in us, and the things outside of us, which
cause them, and between our thought of a
thing and the thing itself. We distinguish
between uttering a cry and hearing it when
we utter it ; between the noise a thing makes
and the thing which makes it. But the
animal and the infant draw none of these
distinctions. To them the world is ' nice ',
' nasty ', ' horrible ', ' strange ', ' enraging ',
or ' familiar ', not ' blue ', ' cold ', ' swift ',
' soft ', ' loud ', ' large ', or ' heavy '. In
fact the mind's first classifications are
emotional rather than objective, and the
first classification of all is doubtless into
' satisfactory ' and ' unsatisfactory '—in
respect of particular needs. So when a
social animal utters a danger cry the others
take to flight merely because the situation
has suddenly become ' fearful '. If we suppose any more complex mental goings-on

[1] There is an influential school of Philosophy, that of Bergson,
which would have us recur, as far as may be, to the more primitive use, to gain thereby a more intimate sense of reality. Cf.
Karin Stephen, *The Misuse of Mind*, 1922, p. 42.

in them we shall be misinterpreting their behaviour. Similarly, when the infant hears its mother speaking kindly, the situation merely becomes ' comfortable ', and its bubbling reply is merely part of this comfortableness ; just as the flight is part of the fearfulness. The contrast drawn by the adult between the situation and the response in such cases only arises much later, and for the animal perhaps never.

The danger and other social cries of animals can be regarded as primitive names, if we are careful to remember how unlike our own mental processes the animal's are. And what they name is not any specific feature of the situation but the whole thing. At the same time the animal does not regard the cry as a name, as a separate part even, of the situation. It is inextricably part of the whole state of affairs even when he utters it himself. This may help us to understand how it is that children, savages, and even men eminent in the world of scholarship, so strangely and so persistently proceed as though the name were part of the thing—a tendency which is still exerting an evil influence upon thought.[1]

[1] Cf. the author's forthcoming *Word Magic* (supplementing *The Meaning of Meaning*, Chapter II), for detailed evidence of this tendency and this influence.

The Child's Conquest of Speech. We gain firmer ground as we pass from speculations to the actual observable behaviour of the savage and the child. The infant's first articulated words, his *mámá*, for example, should be regarded not as names, but more as single word sentences analogous to the adult's commands or appeals. They are specialized cries for help, and are entirely of an expressive character springing directly out of the infant's original needs. Thus they are not very far removed from the exiled chimpanzee's appeals to his companions. But, as a rule, about the middle of the second year of life, a change takes place. A sudden increase in vocabulary combines with a thirst for names.[1] The child makes what has been described as the most important discovery of his life, namely the discovery that things have names. Naturally he jumps to the conclusion that everything has a name, a conclusion which sometimes causes perplexity to his parents ; and from this he goes on to treat his former appeal-

[1] In his work on *The Symbolic Process*, and its integration in children (1928), Chapter vii, Professor J. F. Markey makes a special study of the use of ' personal ' symbols. It is worth noting that a four-year-old may be linguistically active for more than 11½ hours in a 12 hour day, speaking as many as 15,000 words (1,000 different) or 20 words per minute.

words as names, to regard the name as part of the thing, to invent names for things on the ground of a resemblance between the thing as it appears to him and the name, to transfer names to other things which for him are similar, and to combine names already acquired into new names for new and more complex objects. Even general words such as ' this ' or ' one ' or ' make ' get used freely at a very early age.

Imitation. In all this eager and triumphant activity in which the child achieves what often seems to be the greatest intellectual performance of his whole lifetime, we can see clearly the dominant need which is at work. It is his need to escape from his former state of helplessness and to extend his dominion over the world. His main method in this progressive conquest is imitation, and we may, perhaps, best consider here this important feature of behaviour.

There is no necessity to invoke a special instinct for imitation. The connection between hearing a word, not as a mere noise but as an articulate sound, and pronouncing it is very close. The nervous centres concerned are in intimate connection. Whenever the child utters a word, he immediately hears it, and, as we have suggested, it is doubtful whether the young infant makes any distinction between them. The closeness of this connection is shown also by the extraordinary precocity of some children in singing. Erwin Nyiregyházi, for example, the Hungarian boy prodigy, began to imitate singing before he was one year old, and could correctly reproduce melodies before he could speak.[1] The same is reported of Handel.

The Dominion of Society. It will be evident that the acquisition of language is not only an extension of the child's dominion over the world, but also an extension of society's dominion over him. He is forced thereby into closer conformity with already established ways of regarding the world, not only because the wishes of adults can now take a more intimate hold upon him, but because automatically his mind takes over the traditional naming patterns.

Man's dependence upon tradition and upon his membership of a society has led some psychologists to conceive of society as a

[1] G. Révész, *The Psychology of a Musical Prodigy* (1925), p. 7. For a survey of the many curious sidelights thrown by the study of music on psychology see *The Effects of Music* (1927), edited by Max Schoen.

power or force outside of man. If we pay sufficient attention to the ways in which parents and elders influence the child, through language and otherwise, and to the ways in which men influence one another, there is no occasion for such vague speculations. Group or social psychology is the psychology of men in groups or societies. Change a man's group and you change him, but a great deal of confusion reigns among psychologists upon this point.[1] It is a common practice to write of the 'group mind' as though this were something analogous to the individual mind. But we should be clear that it is merely a handy term for a system of individual minds in more or less close interaction. To conceive of it as a 'super-soul', floating outside all the individual minds of the members of the group, is a concession to mental laziness. At present the large and important French school of sociologists influenced by Durkheim is especially prone to this temptation.

The Virtues and Drawbacks of Language. We may regard our linguistic heritage

---

[1] Occasionally, however, as in the case of Dr Burrow's *The Social Basis of Consciousness* (1927), the sympathetic reader can extract something of value from attempts to deal with 'group' difficulties.

both as an immense advantage and, on a smaller scale, as a calamity. When we consider how impotent any single mind would be to make for itself a picture of reality one thousandth part as adequate as that to which language leads us, we see the advantages. The discoverer of the auxiliary verb, of the preposition, and of the definite article should have their portraits, could they be painted, in every school. Needless to say, no such heroes ever existed ; these mighty instruments arose much as our hands gradually became free for general purposes. Yet there is another side to this endowment. At many points language badly misrepresents the world as we know it. All current languages embody in their grammar and vocabulary an outlook upon the world which is passing away. The fact that we are forced to use nouns for what are essentially happenings rather than things (as when we say ' an emotion ', ' a perception ', ' a thought ', instead of an emotional, a perceptual, or a ratiocinative event) is an example. The struggle which psychology is having now to rid itself of a false ' atomism ' and to arrive at ' dynamic ' conceptions is primarily a struggle against a bad legacy in language.

Innumerable other examples could be given. But language has still other drawbacks than this of smuggling inappropriate ideas into our minds while we are too young to protect ourselves. It is the vehicle of tradition in more than intellectual matters. Far too many of our moral attitudes come to us unscrutinized and without proper criticism through language alone. Consider those two prodigious engines of moral discipline, the simple words ' good ' and ' bad '. Originally to the child they are equivalent to ' permitted ' and ' not-permitted '. Little by little the problem, " By whom permitted ? " may be faced ; but in the end any such coherent interpretation of the words usually lapses, the higher reaches of the investigation being so obscure, and the mind is left simply with attitudes of acceptance and rejection which the words touch off. The individual has regressed, in other words, into an infantile or animal state ; ' bad ' has become once more merely a danger cry and ' good ' a lure call. Hence when anything is generally alleged to be good or to be bad, the great majority of people in the great majority of their moments react without any view as to what it is that is being said. This nebulosity is a great obstacle in the many cases in which a revaluation of traditional attitudes is made necessary by changed circumstances and increased knowledge.

Interesting psychological results can be obtained by inviting anyone to try, for a while, to avoid certain controversial words and set-phrases in his discourse, or to limit his vocabulary to less than 1,000 words where previously 10,000 had been drawn upon. Nothing reveals more clearly how much we have come to rely on verbal buoys, to keep afloat in the muddy waters of controversy, than an attempt to substitute ' definitions ', in the vocabulary of a different level of communication, for the irritant and nomadic shorthand of current chat. The word-economy of a total vocabulary of (say) 850 scientifically selected fundamental terms provides a unique mental discipline. Such a limited vocabulary, eliminating (from English) both Verbs (as usually understood) and Emotive terms, has at last actually been devised, both for experimental purposes and as a solution of the problem of an International Auxiliary Language.[1]

Many political and pistic (Gk. *pistis*=

[1]See the writer's *Basic English* (4th Edition, 1933), *Debabelization* (2nd Edition, 1934), etc.

' faith ') watchwords, of which illustrations are not needed or might give offence, are good examples of language which has lapsed unobserved into this infantile condition. It would not, perhaps, be an exaggeration to say that half of what passes for current thought on general affairs is not thought at all, but language operated at a merely emotional level.

There need be nothing surprising in this. Apart from his technical pursuits, his hunting, his building, etc., we have seen that primitive man's outlook is not governed by the facts of nature, but by what we regard as superstitious whimsies ; and this level of mental activity has only been transcended at comparatively rare moments in human history, for example in Assyria under Assurbanipal. We have been living on the legacy of these early achievements ever since, as the Renaissance implies ; and if we have carried the task rather further by the advance of science during the last three hundred years, this should not blind us to the precariousness of our hold upon high civilization. Great though the difference may be in ' seeing things as they are ' between the educated adult and the child or the savage, from another point of view it is still too slight.

CHAPTER X

BEHAVIOUR

The Historical Background of Behaviorism. During the last thirty years academic psychology has received a number of salutary shocks. The greatest of these has come from psycho-analysis. Here was a body of mixed observations and doctrine set forth by doctors who paid practically no attention at all to accepted views, who virtually ignored the fact that a science calling itself psychology was already in existence. The orthodox psychologists for some time retaliated by ignoring psycho-analysis. But however little of the *doctrines* of psycho-analysis becomes ultimately accepted, there can be no doubt that the shock has been salutary. A striking example is a confession of the late Dr Rivers, an exceptionally active and well-informed psychologist. Just before the War he helped to draw up a syllabus for a course in psychological medicine. When he came to revise it just after the War he discovered to his astonishment that it included no mention of Instinct.[1] This change of view among orthodox psychologists was due more to the labours of Freud than to anything else.

But to-day the conception of instinct is itself being challenged by none more vigorously than by Watson and the Behaviorists whose views have given a fresh shock—more particularly to American psychology. Other countries have hitherto paid remarkably little attention, perhaps because in Europe sides have already often been taken on what is regarded as in part a religious issue.[2]

The Nature of Observation. The doctrine of Behaviorism can be summed up briefly in two statements: (1) That psychology deals only with what can be observed. (2) That 'consciousness' is a meaningless term. It is worth while to consider each of these statements closely.

When the behaviorist speaks of *observation*

[1] W. H. R. Rivers, *Psychology and Politics* (1923), p. 4. The gradual development of Dr Rivers' views in this and in other connexions can be seen in his three works, *Conflict and Dream* (1923), *Medicine Magic and Religion* (1924), and *Psychology and Ethnology* (1924), which are of interest from another angle in that Dr Rivers was a leading figure in academic psychology throughout the first quarter of the present century.

[2] Cf. the controversies arising out of the doctrines of Hobbes, La Mettrie, Condillac, Bentham, Comte, and G. H. Lewes, for example, as dealt with in Lange's monumental work, *The History of Materialism*.

he means something which can be done by a photographic film or a spring balance just as well as by a human being. What is observed is one event, the observation of it is another ; and what happens is merely that the observed event under suitable conditions is accompanied by the observing event—which varies with it. Thus an observation is simply one form of what is called a ' causal sequence '[1] and any event succeeding and varying with another might, on a behaviorist account, be said to observe it. But the particular observations with which the behaviorist is concerned are events in people, in human observers, which follow other events in other people or in themselves. Now it would appear at first sight that events in people and in ourselves could be divided into two kinds : those which are conscious, or are accompanied by consciousness—as when we hear a noise, have a tooth out, are frightened, lift a heavy weight or deliberately choose between actions ; and those which are not conscious, not accompanied by consciousness—as when by a series of muscular contractions we pass food through the

---

[1] For a clear discussion of modern views of causation Bertrand Russell's *The A B C of Relativity* (1925, uniform with this work), pp. 103-205, may be very profitably consulted.

K

stomach, when we balance ourselves, dilate the pupil, or perform a habitual involuntary gesture. This difference which has nearly always been considered very striking, unmistakable, and fundamental, is denied by strict behaviorists. And this denial is the novel point in their doctrine.

There is, of course, something very unsatisfactory about introspection as a scientific method.[1] There is also the feeling that any adding in of ' conscious ' factors which cannot be measured and do not obey the same laws as the rest of nature must play havoc with all hopes of satisfactory explanations ; and this feeling is justified. An essentially physiological explanation ought not to be eked out by scraps of experience. It should remain physiology. But this is not—and here the Behaviorists made their mistake—the same thing as saying that there can be no study of consciousness or that the study may not provide valuable indications in working out a physiological theory of behaviour. In point of fact, it constantly so serves.

[1] Cf. MacCurdy, *The Psychology of Emotion*, p. 59 : " We all of us introspect to the advantage of our pet theories . . . the most valid material is to be derived from the experience of those who are not trained introspectionists."

But it is one thing to say : " Let us try to describe and explain all human behaviour entirely in terms of interaction between stimulus-situation and response ", and quite another to say : " Let us try to persuade people that they have no consciousness ". The first is of real value, and likely, if it can be carried rather further, to change our views on many points, and possibly to bring out the rôle of consciousness in a new light.

The second is merely waste of time ; and whatever view we may take the controversy cannot be carried very far without a more subtle sense of verbal pitfalls than is generally cultivated.

The Origins of Fear. One of Watson's most interesting observations was that the peculiar and recognizable response which is ordinarily known as fear, " a jump, a start, a respiratory pause followed by more rapid breathing with marked vasomotor changes " (changes in the blood flow, *e.g.*, growing pale), sudden closure of the eye, clutching of hands, puckering of lips, is only elicited in ' new-borns ' by two kinds of stimuli, loud noises, and being suddenly left without support. But as is well known, a normal three-year-old shows fear for a great number of other things. Here is a representative list from Watson : darkness, and all rabbits, rats, dogs, fish, frogs, insects, and mechanical animal toys. Watson's thesis is that all these fears arise because at some time the appearance of a dog, for example, has co-incided with either a loud noise or being knocked over (loss of support). The dog later, when it merely approaches causes the fear, just as the note caused Pavlov's dog's mouth to water. This fear then gets transferred to other situations which the infant groups with it,[1] and so on. Evidently this view has no use for ' instincts ' except in the sense of initial characteristic responses to characteristic situations. But these, as Watson points out, are shown by a boomerang, which when properly thrown behaves quite unlike an ordinary stick. The child would be a very complicated kind of boomerang, and its instincts merely the result of its structure at birth.

Now this, it will be realized, is, if it is correct, an extremely important contribution. Watson finds in children who have not been emotionally conditioned no such fears

---

[1] Thus Albert, eleven months old, who had an (experimentally) conditioned fear of a white rat, showed fear five days later of a rabbit, a dog; a fur coat, cotton wool, but not of bricks.

of dogs or darkness, and if this is established, the prospect of a comparatively fearless humanity is opened up if only we can manage our nurseries aright. There is, however, the possibility that maturation may introduce complications. Even though loud noises and loss of support be the only stimuli which cause fear immediately after birth, it is possible that later on other stimuli come to have the same effect merely through the infant's growth. Maturation certainly plays some part, and some very definite responses only appear at a very late age. The specific sexual responses appearing with adolescence are an obvious instance.

The Unconditioned Emotions. The exact truth in this matter will only be discovered by further experimental research, and Watson is undoubtedly to be congratulated for the part he has played in furthering such experimentation. He has come to consider that the unlearned (unconditioned) beginnings of emotional reactions are three in number. Fear, elicited as above, Rage, elicited by hampering of bodily movements, and Love, elicited by stroking of the skin, tickling, gentle rocking, and patting. Love

responses include " those popularly called
' affectionate ', ' good-natured ', ' kindly ',
. . . as well as the responses we see in adults
between the sexes. They all have a common
origin ".

Watson further points out that since the
same object (say a parent) may in one situation become a conditioned stimulus for fear,
in another for rage, and in another for love,
these three original groups of responses can
easily become complicated through experience.
Only, he does not use the word ' experience '.
To do so would be to link his labours up with
those of more traditional psychologists. His
extremely provoking attitude towards academic psychologists and towards psycho-analysts
alike, amusing and inspiriting though it is
when we realize that his work is likely to
be of great assistance to them and is not in
conflict with theirs, is to be regretted if it
debars them, as it may, from taking due
notice and advantage of it. They have already
shown too often the natural tendency to
reply in kind. It may be suggested that
these very different views and methods are
not irreconcilable. Nothing so readily gives
a beginner in psychology a sense of helplessness and annoyance as the existence of

violently opposed views [1] which he more often than not rightly suspects to be mere verbal variants.

[1] The reader who desires to test his ingenuity in sifting disagreement as to facts from differences of formulation cannot do better than study *The Battle of Behaviorism* (Watson-McDougall debate). Similar material in a closely related field is provided by *Man not a Machine* (Rignano) and *Man a Machine* (Needham) ; while a still more curious example of modern debating methods is provided by a fourth volume (uniform with the above, in the *Psyche* Miniatures) entitled *Culture : the Diffusion Controversy*, a Symposium.

CHAPTER XI

LOOKING INWARDS

BOUVARD and Pécuchêt, in the great novel by
Flaubert, resolved to take up psychology.
The goal of psychology, they read, is to study
the facts which take place " in the bosom of
the self " ; these are discovered by introspection. " And for a fortnight, after breakfast regularly, they hunted about at random
in their minds, hoping to make notable
discoveries, and made none and were much
surprised."

The Elusiveness of Consciousness.
They had reason to be surprised, for it is
indeed odd that introspection tells us so little.
If the old metaphysical view, that the known
and the knower must be alike, were sound,
our own minds should be the most certain
objects of our knowledge. Yet they are
to-day perhaps the least certain. The most
mysterious thing in the universe to man is
at present himself, his own mind and its

nature. It has not always been so. In the ages of faith, the Dark Ages, as the historians have called them, the outside world seemed much more mysterious than man. Thus he tried to explain it in terms of himself. He either made it a stage on which the drama of his own life was enacted, a thing with no further interest of its own, or he pictured it as being animated and guided somewhat after the fashion of himself. The balance has changed since then. Nowadays his tendency is to conceive himself as far as possible in terms of his knowledge of the outer world.

It is curious to reflect that the things which man best understands are on the whole the things which least concern him. He can predict the movements of the planets, but not the weather, he has fathomed the deep sea, but cannot measure his own desires, he knows more about beer than about his blood . . . and at the heart of all his knowledge is a mystery, namely how he gets it. This last problem we shall discuss later. Here we have a simpler task, to describe *from within* what conscious life is like, basing our account upon the facts which are always accessible to everyone.

The reason why Bouvard and Pécuchêt made no discoveries was that they asked no definite questions. It is only by *interrogating* consciousness that we get any light upon it. It will be well to begin by drawing up a list of the principal questions we propose to raise in the order in which we shall raise them :

(1) What is the Self ?

(2) What kind of a thing is an experience ?

(3) What are the essential aspects of experience ?

The answers to these questions must inevitably be tentative. The value of studying them lies not in the answers which we obtain, but in the insight into our nature which results from the inquiry.

The Distorting Influence of Language. Throughout this undertaking we must beware of three allied dangers. In the first place, language was not developed with a view to this account. Not only is there a bad shortage of words for the task, but such words as we are compelled to use are ill fitted to it, and distort the account unless we watch them closely and do not take them too much at their face value. Language was developed to describe (at the common-sense level) what we see or hear, not to describe seeing or hearing. It is a distorting influence here not only as a vocabulary, but as a syntax. For example, it is natural to say ' I have a thought '. But that suggests a fact analogous to ' I have a penny ', whereas what it really stands for would be better put by saying " A thinking is happening in me " ; but even here ' in ' and ' me ' are misleading. And when we talk of ' ideas ', ' sensations ', or ' pleasures ' the case, as we shall see, is worse still. Language, in fact, is not only a means by which we hide our thoughts from other people ; it is a veil which helps to hide our own lives from ourselves.

Hypotheses and Abstractions. The second danger is no less insidious. It comes from the great difficulty of distinguishing here between our hypotheses and the facts these hypotheses were introduced to explain. The Self, strange as it may appear, is such an hypothesis ; so are, more evidently, the Will, the Memory, the Intelligence, the Instincts, and the Unconscious. And in fact most of the terms of psychology stand for hypotheses, not for facts. The facts are there all the while, they make up our lives, but it is impossible to weave them together into any intelligible system without some hypotheses. The trouble is that we easily mistake the hypotheses for the facts. When we reflect upon our experience they tend to come between us and the facts.

The third danger is one on which Bergson has particularly insisted. When we analyse an experience theoretically we often find it convenient to suppose it built up out of certain elements in certain combinations. For example, much psychology has proceeded successfully on the assumption that *sensations* are the basic elements out of which all experience is compounded. An amazing amount of detailed information about our perception of nature has been achieved by the aid of this assumption. So that it comes as a shock to be forced to ask : " Do we ever have sensations ? " None the less this question must not only be asked but be decided in the negative.

The Conscious Subject or Self. With these dangers in view we may proceed. What is the first obvious and overwhelming fact about our ordinary experience ? It is that it seems *to belong to us*, to be the experience of a self. We do not find isolated bits of experience belonging to nobody. All experience seems to be attached to, to be part of, a system of experiences which we call a person or say belongs to a person. In fact, it is impossible to describe a complete concrete bit of experience without bringing in either a proper name or a personal pronoun. We find experience always organized into personal histories.

The Dynamic View of the Mind. It is important to realize, in spite of language, that the mind is not a thing, but an activity. We are so accustomed to thinking in terms of things like bricks, loaves, boots, atoms, and electrons, which, if they change at all, do so in such crude fashions and affect one another in such simple ways, that to conceive of experience as a system of energies whose changes bear very little analogy to the changes in such ' material objects ' is difficult. Those possessing some slight acquaintance with, for example, elementary electrical theory, will have an advantage here. For they will be less exposed to the danger of conceiving the matter too crudely.

A vocabulary of ' tensions ', ' stresses ',

' impulses ', ' currents ', ' tendencies ', and ' flows ' is far more adequate in describing experiences than one of ' sensation ', ' percepts ', ' ideas ', ' concepts ,' and ' images '. This is what the assertion that experience is dynamic, that the mind is an activity, amounts to. These traditional psychological terms are in fact a serious obstacle to a real understanding. They suggest too much that consciousness is a kind of shop window containing these various items in various arrangements with a mysterious factory in the background turning out the products displayed. These images, ideas, etc., are, however, not products, but *processes*. What we observe when we introspect is the working of the factory itself. An image or an idea is a change, a redistribution of energies. Hence the peculiar fluidity of consciousness passing away from us always like a stream. And if we think of our experiences as like waves or eddies rather than like the flowing water or bits of stick passing down the stream, we shall come nearer to an adequate conception.

Disturbance and Recovery of Equilibrium. One further general character of experience must be noted before we go on to consider it in more detail. This concerns the way, in general, that these changes come about. We have already hinted that an experience only becomes an ' object ' for consciousness if it needs in some way to be dealt with. And we may take the ' subject ' to be the rest of the mind, which is called upon to deal with it. The important point here, important on any view of the self, is that experience is initiated through the need for the mind to deal with a situation—that is, to make a new adaptation. Our everyday psychological language is full of phrases suggesting the importance of this fact. ' To attend to ' something means ordinarily to try to put it right, or to put ourselves right with regard to it. To ' be concerned with ' has a similar sense, and so has to ' be interested in ' (literally, to interest is to make a difference).

If we ask ourselves why on any occasion we are having one kind of experience rather than another we find that it is because in this experience we are dealing with a situation, setting ourselves right with regard to it or setting it right with regard to us, or attempting to do so. This is true whether we take extensive and lengthy experiences (a courtship or legal action, for example) or brief and restricted experiences (a moment of introspection). In every case what is happening is essentially an attempt to restore equilibrium to a system of activities which has been disturbed. The disturbance may come from without; it may be due to a smell of burning which *disturbs our equanimity* as regards the safety of our dwelling. We sniff, set down our glass, get up, and take whatever steps we can think of to make sure all is well. Only thereby can the system of impulses which has been disturbed come to rest again. Or the disturbance may come from within: we remember suddenly that we have not posted a letter, and the uneasy feeling that ensues drives us out to do so.

The Ultimate Modes of Consciousness. The threefold distinction which almost all psychologists have made between knowing, feeling, and striving (or cognition, affection, and conation, as they call them) can be easily made out in nearly every experience.[1] It is a knowing of, or thinking about, something; it is pleasurable or unpleasant; and it is a striving towards something. Each is

[1] The importance of this union is well stressed in Paulhan's *The Laws of Feeling* (1929).

a distinct kind of consciousness. Striving (motor consciousness), for example, is not to be reduced to cognition, though many psychologists have identified it with kinæsthetic sensations. We must beware, however, of the temptation to regard them as isolable. Any one of them may lapse so as to be hardly, if at all, present, and there are perhaps states of mind in which they are not distinguishable ; but we do not find processes which are purely cognitive, purely affective, or purely conative, any more than we find moving bodies which have no mass, or lines in nature which have no breadth. When the psychologist says that they are irreducible he means that none of them can be described in terms of the others.

Only by treating cognition in isolation was it possible to construct philosophical systems on so-called 'sense-data'. Psychology has shown that the simplest of all experiences is a highly complex *process* ; and this result is of fundamental consequence for our general speculative outlook on the world. To put it shortly, what have for centuries been regarded as the foundations of all our knowledge have given way, and no one is any the worse for it.

L

Shock. But what exactly is the difference between something which we do and something which merely happens to us? It is clear enough sometimes to introspection. Compare the experience of looking at a picture with that of having a tooth drawn, or listening to music with being in a boiler factory or a metropolis. The difference is that we *respond* to the picture or the music ; to the shock we react. In a response our perceptions are steps we take as a result of stimulation, steps towards adjustment. If the adjustment is easy and smooth, but not so easy as to be automatic and stereotyped, we feel pleased ; if it is difficult or fails, we feel displeasure. The whole conscious experience in either case is controlled by the precise condition of the new poise towards which we are tending. Consider the needle of a compass. There is a certain position at which the magnetic forces acting upon it are in equipoise. If we disturb it, there ensue wagglings, steps through which it returns to a position of rest. By a metaphor which is not too strained we can say that it is seeking this position. Now picture the needle geared up to a motor and driven round and round. This roughly represents what happens to us in the dentist's chair, in the boiler factory, or under the sand-bag of the apache. Instead of responding, according to the laws of our own structure, to the disturbance which has set us waggling, instead of dealing with the situation, the situation is dealing with us.

From this brief indication the reader will be able to see how a detailed account would run. The essential point is that in perception what happens is governed by the end-state of poise towards which we are tending, whereas, in sensation, on the comparatively rare occasions on which it occurs, all possibility of tending to an equipoise is set aside by the violent, paralysing shock of the occurrence.

In all introspection we must remember that what appears to be happening when we look inwards is different from what happens when we are not so engaged ; and also that events of the mind hide behind one another. Thus our general organic sensibility due to the state of our body as a whole and known by the name of cenesthesia (Gk. *koinos=* common ; and *aisthesis=*sensation) is always colouring our consciousness, but to take note of it in introspection is extraordinarily difficult. We are much more likely to describe it as a peculiar peacefulness or vividness about the landscape, or a singular glare in the light or stuffiness in the air, than as what it really is.

Pleasure-Unpleasure. Passing now to the pleasure-unpleasure aspect, the *affective* aspect as it is called, we may note first how central this seems in all experience. Probably this is largely an illusion. Pleasure and unpleasure are products of our activities rather than their sources. Two questions arise for consideration : (1) Do pleasure and unpleasure make up the whole of the affective aspect ? and (2) What exactly is their —evidently close—connection with striving ? As to (1) it seems at first sight natural to bring emotional characters of experience under this heading. Fear, disgust, anger, and love may seem at least to contain specific modifications of consciousness with as good a right to be classed among affective phenomena as pleasure or unpleasure. But when we look more closely these emotional characters turn out to be composite. We cannot reduce pleasure and unpleasure either to awareness or to striving or to a blend of the two ; but we can reduce fear to a union of awareness, unpleasure and conscious striving, and its peculiar character is given it by what we are aware of, how we are striving, and, as a rule, unpleasure. (2) External observations also corroborate introspection as regards the second question. Pleasure and unpleasure are very intimately connected with the course of striving, with its progress towards ' satisfactory ' or ' unsatisfactory ' stage. Success seems always to be pleasant, and failure unpleasant, but the success or failure may be local merely, as we need hardly point out ; and a great success, though intensely pleasant, may be from the point of view of the whole organism, the whole history of the mind, a disaster. So it is with the ecstasies of the drug addict.

Pains. Pains need a word of elucidation perhaps. They are usually unpleasant but not always ; and some people enjoy playing with a not too sensitive tooth. It is best to distinguish them sharply from the unpleasure which ordinarily accompanies them and to regard them as a special class of perceptions, a class which has for obvious biological reasons a precedence normally over most other perceptions since they arise for the most part from what are called *nocuous* stimuli, stimuli likely to lead to damage of the tissues. But as in our early example ot the climber attacked by a wasp, and as many surprising abnormal phenomena show, pain may lose this precedence. In hypnotic conditions, even major operations can be performed without the patient showing any signs of pain, and there is the classic story of a cheerful and corpulent politician, who in an election crisis calmly bit off his damaged finger as though it were the most natural thing in the world to do.

Enjoyment and Absorption. Our general analysis can be applied to every kind of experience. The states of enjoyment to which the term Beauty is probably best restricted show more clearly than any others the reconciliation of the most varied impulses in a balanced integral experience (synæsthesis).[1]

Usually, in ordinary life, we are not a single stream, but a welter of many semi-independent streams. We may be adding up figures, watching a neighbour, and thinking of what we shall do later in the evening simultaneously. Several separately disturbed systems are tending independently to their

---

[1] For an analysis, by the author and others, of the many very different uses of the term Beauty and of their psychological basis, see *The Foundations of Æsthetics*, second edition, 1925, London and New York ; also the *Encyclopaedia Britannica*, 13th edition (1926 Supplementary Volume), where this analysis appears in its historical setting.

end-states. When there is only one such process going on we say we are *absorbed* by what we are doing. When there are too many such separate disturbances or when the settlement of one interferes with that of the others we complain of distraction. In deep absorption, as is evident from the story of the Mysore mathematician who tied a cobra round his neck in mistake for a cravat, a change in the general situation which would ordinarily cause deep disturbance passes apparently unnoticed. What happens in such cases is difficult to decide. It is often alleged that such changes are *always* noticed, unconsciously. The possibility of sometimes recovering them from memory, by hypnosis or other special means, as in psycho-analysis, is the evidence for this view. It is not very strong evidence, however, for we more often never remember them and they have no observable effect upon us whatever.

The Limits of Consciousness. What probably happens in the majority of cases is that we do consciously notice the change, but, since for the moment it has no significance for us, we do nothing further about it. Thus our response to it is extremely brief and does not initiate further disturbances

as it would if we were *attending*. For our
deeper disturbances are always due to prior
responses to shallower disturbances. When
we recognize something, this recognition
(itself a response to a disturbance) may,
like the fuse of a shell, throw much more
important systems into turmoil. But in
deep absorption the linkage between our
systems of impulses is impaired, for all
systems save those which are already active.

Interests may be unconscious as well as
conscious. As to why some are and others
are not we know as yet very little. Sometimes an interest seems to be unconscious
because consciousness of it would be unpleasant. Yet many unpleasant interests are
conscious. This part of psychology, to which
we return later (Chapter XIV), is as yet
comparatively in its infancy. To consider
it we have to pass outside the bounds of
introspection, which are beginning to appear
curiously and significantly restricted. Our
minds certainly are far larger than our
normal consciousness, but it may be remarked
that this has been discovered chiefly through
special means (hypnosis and psycho-analysis)
which have enabled the bounds of introspection to be extended.

CHAPTER XII

LOOKING OUTWARDS

Our Knowledge of the External World.
We are apt to regard our knowledge of the
outside world as a matter of course, and to
think that things can hardly help being
much as we perceive them. But here again
psychology is unsettling. We are not nearly
in such close contact as we suppose with even
the things we seem to know best—our chairs,
our motor-cycles, our friends. We have seen
(Chapter III) how stimuli falling upon special
sense organs at the surface of the body cause
impulses to be volleyed in along the afferent
neurones leading to reception and co-ordinating centres ; and how they there compete
for the discharge of these centres and thus for
a share in still more intricate transactions
of the association circuits. And in the
chapters which followed we saw how far
from passive we are in our perceptions, and
the extent to which what we see depends
upon our needs and interests. We have

now to look rather more closely at all this with a view to discovering, if we may, how much of the world is really there before us as we ordinarily think it and how much of it is merely a reflection of ourselves.

Illusions of Sight and Touch. Certain well-known illusions show clearly how complex

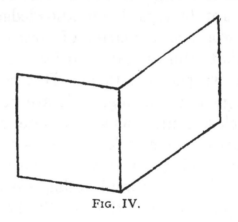

FIG. IV.

our perceptual processes are even when they seem simple. Bend a visiting card or a small piece of smooth paper so that it will stand upright like a half-open book upon the tablecloth (Fig. IV), and gaze at it with one eye. You can see it either as if opening towards you or away from you. (Notice also the ways in which the colours tend to become more noticeable in the 'unreal' position).

Or look with both eyes at Fig. V. It can be seen either as one cube or as another, or as a series of boxes with the tops or the sides off, or as a flat design.

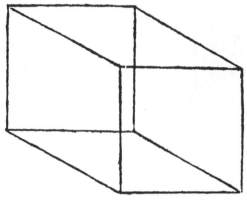

FIG. V.

The Monument-Gateway ambiguity (Fig. VI) is still more striking. By gazing steadily it can be seen either as a solid or as an opening ; while the staircase below it can also be seen as an overhanging cornice. In Figure VII the warriors, though drawn the same height, appear, through the illusion of perspective, to be one taller than the other. The alternating relief is related to the phenomena of blood pressure, whereas the perspective illusion is probably due to the

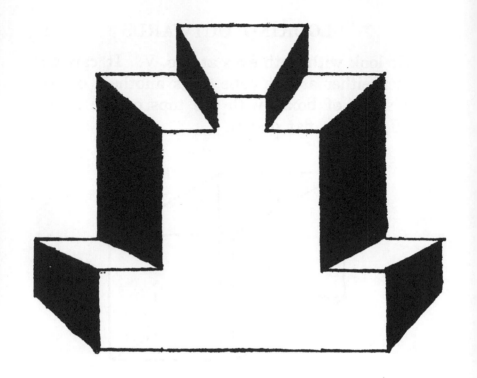

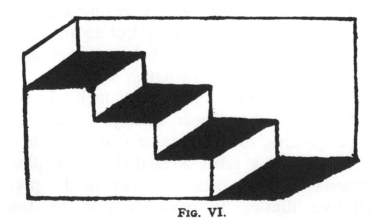

FIG. VI.

expectation of ocular convergence which produces a giant in the middle distance. To

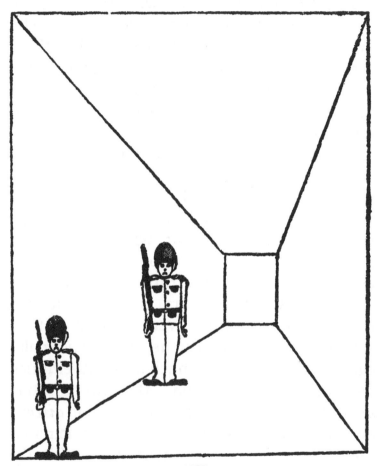

FIG. VII.

take a different sense, try to hold a walking-
stick vertically with your eyes shut and
your head bent well over to one side, or cross

two fingers and touch them with a pencil placed between them.

Eye-movements. It will repay us to consider eye-movements a little more closely. Without the experimental work and without the neurological evidence, we should never have realized what an astonishing amount they do for us, and how much of our world depends upon them.

Consider dizziness, for example. This seems to us merely an odd and unpleasant experience to be avoided when possible. Yet it is but the exaggerated or disturbed working of a mechanism without which we should never know where we are or where anything else is. Whenever we turn about, a small apparatus within the ears, containing a fluid resembling sea-water,[1] very like a set of spirit-levels and known as the semicircular canals, takes note of it much as a half-emptied flask in our pocket would. But this agitation in itself tells us nothing. It does not *directly* give rise to perceptions ; the semicircular canals have little direct connection with the cortex of the cerebrum. And yet our sense of orientation, our knowledge of which way

---

[1] This, together with the salinity of our blood-plasma, is part of the evidence for man's aquatic ancestry in the remote past.

we are facing, and our whole left-and-right-turn consciousness, undoubtedly do depend upon what happens in these semicircular canals. They tell us indirectly by a reflex provocation of turning movements of the eyes to right and left. It is these eye-movements which tell us when we turn, and without them we have no sense of turning. The dizzy man, when he shuts his eyes, feels as though *he* was turning ; if he opens them the things he sees seem to spin round, but the other way.

This extraordinary indirectness with which we perceive what is happening is paralleled almost everywhere in perception. A pinch or a stab with a pin might seem to be given directly just where it is ; but not so. It has to be found, so to speak, and its localization depends upon the reflexes which it sets up ; if these are deranged it becomes misplaced.

Recognition. But these are mere superficial complexities in the mechanism of perception. Let us go a step deeper. Consider how we perceive forms which are familiar to us. Something is put into our hand ; we perceive it instantly to be a key without any process of exploring it with the fingers. Certain injuries to the brain make this impossible, but we may still be able by exploratory movements to make out its shape and form without being able to recognize it *as* a key. And other injuries produce the converse effect. We can tell that it is a key, yet cannot work out what the shape is. This last is the really puzzling instance. We can find many parallels in normal life. There are people, there are expressions, there are situations which we recognize instantly, yet if we try to work out what it is that distinguishes them from other people, expressions or situations, we fail altogether to get a satisfactory explanation. Of course in such cases we may make mistakes, and probably far more often than we suppose. Yet how a chair seen from a new angle is recognized at once as that same chair, is the fundamental question in perception.

It is natural to suppose that something, its colour or some detail of shape, is the cause of the identification ; and this no doubt is usually the case. But the detail itself may be presented to us at an angle from which we have never before perceived it. The more difficult problem is how this *new* aspect may be instantly responded to, in spite of its difference from all the aspects which we have formerly beheld. It seems clear that the mind (or a co-ordination centre in the brain, if we prefer so to put it) responds not only to stimuli which it has already received, but thereafter to a certain range of stimuli. When these other stimuli closely resemble the original, this is not surprising. But in many cases the set of aspects by which we instantly recognize a thing are extraordinarily varied. A coin seen with the rim or the flat side showing is very different. Yet we recognize even unfamiliar things from new aspects without difficulty.

Sign-interpretation. This fact, that we recognize what we have never seen, is not difficult to explain if we take account of the ways in which our outlook upon the world has developed. The adult has been watching things move and studying their systematic transformations of shape most of his life. Thus as regards most objects a very wide range of shapes have become equivalent for him ; they are aspects of one object. When he sees a new object, the trace or disposition left in him is not a single isolated pattern of the sensory stimulation, but a setting, ready if need be to respond to an immense variety of patterns—most of those, in fact, into which

M

this pattern can be transformed by movements of the object. This influence of experience explains why the expert—the entomologist or the seaman, for example—is so much more quick and accurate than the amateur in interpreting professional signs.

Most recognition is an extremely complicated performance. We have seen already how interest affects it. But innumerable other factors also play a part. The whole situation must be taken into account if we are to understand recognition. For example, a stimulus which in war-time we should interpret rightly as a sign of an air raid we may equally rightly after the cessation of hostilities interpret as an earthquake. Yet in neither case need we make any conscious reference to the international situation. The general circumstances bar out all but a relatively small number of the possibilities, and our recognition is a choice between those responses which are left. Sufficient attention is rarely given to these wider factors in interpretation by those who concentrate on the elementary problems of recognition.

General Consequences. But on any possible view of recognition in the light of the facts and analyses now at our disposal

our account of interpretation in the wider
sense, the sense in which it is relevant to
current speculation on the reality of the
external world, must make psychology the
key to the riddle of the universe. To some,
indeed, psychological study seems to yield
conclusive evidence that the further we go
the less we shall know. " We can never
solve the so-called world-riddle because what
seem riddles to us are merely the contradictions we have ourselves created," says Havelock Ellis. " We make our own world ;
when we have made it awry we can remake
it approximately truer. . . . Man lives by
imagination." And Vaihinger has urged that
the contradictions which thought endeavours
to resolve are actually essential to its successful operation. In any case, he holds, we can
never free ourselves from psychological
accretions ; for just as the digestive system
breaks up the matter which it received,
mixes it with its own juices and so makes
it suitable for assimilation in the practical
interests of the organism, " so the psyche
envelops the thing perceived with categories
which it has developed out of itself ".

Our intellectual chyme and chyle would,
for those who accept this account, be no

guide whatever to the physical happenings outside our skin, since perception is not even a process of assimilation on the causal view ; nothing of the external stimulus (usually a form of vibration) is actually taken in by the receptors.

Fictions in Modern Physics. This insistence on the psychological foundations of our theories of the external world receives frequent support from the utterances of the most respected modern physicists.

For some, the tendency of the mind to select only the permanent, reinforced as it is by the analytic influence of language, has seemed of necessity to render any scientific account of the universe arbitrary. And the theory of relativity has much to say about the mental factor in scientific explanation. " All through the physical world ", according to Professor Eddington, " runs an unknown content, which must really be the stuff of our consciousness. . . . We have found that where science has progressed the farthest, the mind has but regained from nature that which the mind has put into nature." And again (1929) : " Consciousness is not sharply defined but fades into subconsciousness ; and beyond that we must

postulate something indefinite but yet con-
tinuous with our own mental nature. This I
take to be the world stuff."[1] Psychology
must come to the rescue--if it can !

One of the greatest thinkers of modern
times, Jeremy Bentham (1748-1832), understood this most clearly, and he published
over a century ago an analysis of the fictions
with which we people the world, chiefly as
a result of our misunderstandings of linguistic
psychology. His work, however, has been
completely neglected, and credit has been
given to others for a partial rediscovery of
his point of view, with little realization of
the part played by language in generating
the entities in question. There is no better
introduction to the most abstruse problems
on which psychology has just begun to
throw light than a careful study of Bentham's
Theory of Fictions.

Moreover, it is not sufficiently stressed by
historians of philosophy that on a systematic
reclassification of the subject-matter of the
sciences not only ' solipsists ' (Lat. *solus,
ipse*=alone, myself) but the majority of
those who in the past have called themselves
Idealists, maintaining that to be known is
to be " in the mind " or an " invention of

[1] *The Nature of the Physical World*, 1928, p. 280.

mind ", have in reality endeavoured still further to extend the scope of a possible psychology, though without themselves actually embarking on its details.

The Human Equation. Whatever we may think of such speculations, the general question raised at the beginning of this chapter—How far do our ways of perceiving the world really tell us what it is like and how far do they only tell us what we are like ?—is one which the psychologist will ultimately be called upon to answer. It may be that the physicist, in reacting against an uncritical account of ' matter ', will be found to have gone too far. But in any case the sort of difficulties we have been considering are essential preliminaries to that answer, remote though the issue may have appeared to those who approach the subject for the first time. The reorientations and revaluations which have given rise to psychology as a serious branch of science have occurred in the lifetime of many who are still engaged in its development. It is still premature to speak of final conclusions when we are only beginning to learn to think.

It is surprising how little the psychology of imagination has as yet been utilized in

the service of physics. Our powers of conceiving the world in other aspects than
those suggested by foraging and engineering
have hardly been explored at all. Writers
like Lewis Carroll, Fournier d'Albe, Helen
Keller, Henshaw Ward, Nicod, Haldane, and
Fox have, in different ways, no less than the
physicists we have mentioned, made a remarkable beginning. But the windows which
might be opened on the world by a full study
of animal, primitive, and abnormal psychology (cf. Chapter XVII) are still for the
most part darkened by prejudice and ignorance. At any rate, it is clear that for some
time to come a chief task of psychology is
that of demarcation ;   for, as we shall see
when dealing with emotion, we constantly
project our feelings as well as our constructions
into the outer world. Psychology can point
to the difference between the infant and the
trained observer in all branches of natural
knowledge, and it can describe this difference
fairly definitely. The child, as we saw, fails
comparatively to separate the factors in
perception introduced by his desires from the
factors which the external situation supplies.
The pursuit of truth is the slow weeding out
of the desire factors. One of the chief ways

in which it is done is through the distinction between means and ends. To remain unbiased in the manipulation of means is often indispensable if we are to attain the ends desired. Thus the scientist learns not to cook his evidence if he wishes to prove his conclusion. Even the astronomer has a ' personal equation ' to eliminate, before he regards his observations as objective.

When all desire has been discounted we may still, as Vaihinger maintains, be left in our view of nature with a distortion due to the instrument (the mind) which is viewing it. For this distortion the only possible correction is an exact knowledge of how the mind works. In other words, psychology must criticize itself. Our account of the mind must at least be such that the mind could know about itself. And probably the desire-bias of which we have spoken is stronger in psychology than in any other science. We may well be such as we should hate to think we are. For some of these biases, however, we are learning to allow, chiefly as a result of the discoveries of the psycho-analysts. But we shall be more ready to discuss their findings when we have considered how we think and the nature of our emotions.

CHAPTER XIII

HOW WE THINK

Ideas. Thinking, according to Babbitt, would consist in getting hold of, getting rid of, arranging, and working out ideas; but just what ideas are is a point which he leaves vague. It is this point which we have now to consider.

One account which is of great historical significance regards ideas as images. Ideas obviously *represent* in some way the things that they are *of*; and since images are the mental events which most plainly represent things, this view had much in its favour. But it breaks down if we have to admit that many people think without images, that even when images occur they may be quite irrelevant and accidental, and that they tend to appear chiefly after the thinking has got into difficulties. Words and images are invaluable *helps* in thinking; they are not necessary to it.

Images. It is important to realize that individuals differ enormously in the type of image they employ. One man will use predominantly visual images (though many who think they are visualizers are really making use of eye-movements) ; another, auditory ; another, kinæsthetic—*i.e.*, images of movements of the limbs and trunk. Indeed, every sensation may have its corresponding imagery, and organic sensations, which, as we shall see, play a great part in emotion, may also be represented. What are sometimes referred to as verbal images are of course only images of words and not a special type of image ; they may be of three kinds, visual (as when we see a printed or written word in the mind's eye), auditory (as when we hear an imagined voice), or motor (as when we have an image corresponding to the sensations which accompany speech). It is of little use to appeal to a person of a primarily auditory type by means of diagrams or metaphors deriving from vision. All forms of imagery tend to be heightened at the onset of sleep, and this may be connected with the fact that vivid imagery is more frequent in childhood. The vividness of dream images may be a result of regression or a return to the state of our early years (of. Chapters VIII and XV).

But the rest of the conscious happenings which take place in thinking are far less easy to describe : a sense of the end to be reached, a sense of the direction in which the thought is moving, a sense of orientation, of our whereabouts, senses of novelty and familiarity and of reality, of ease and difficulty, of the relations between our thoughts, and a variety of attitudes towards the stages of the thinking, towards the problem and the answer. To all these imagery has often been regarded as providing a key.

Representation. It is certainly tempting to suppose that the only way in which one thing (a mental event, for example) can represent another (a lobster, perhaps) is by resembling it. Accordingly, many philosophers have made resemblance, identity of structure, fundamental for the explanation of how our ideas come to be *of* things. " We make for ourselves pictures of facts ", says Wittgenstein in his famous *Tractatus Logico-Philosophicus*. " The picture is a model of reality." But is this resemblance really necessary ? The instances we gave in the last chapter of the indirect ways in which we take cognizance of space are enough to make it very doubtful. The movement of a klaxon down the street and the reflexes through which we notice it seem to have no very obvious identity of structure. And in fact the more closely we study the processes by which we perceive things the less plausible is it to suppose that they are necessarily reflections or models of the things. Yet in some sense they represent these things. What is this sense? The answer seems to be that our mental events represent things not through being models or reflections of them, but by being the effects in us of contact with them.

The point at issue may appear a little obscure, but the question is really very simple and, like many simple questions, it is of fundamental importance. What is the link between our minds and the world in virtue of which our thoughts are about the world, are thoughts *of* things, not merely isolated happenings in our minds? In other words, *what is knowing?* If we can answer this question, the rest of our account of thinking is an easier matter. For thinking is merely the testing and manipulation of knowledge in the service of our purposes.

The simplest form of thinking about things

is perceiving them, and this we have already described above. The next most obvious form is imagining them, through reproducing the mental events which occurred in perception. In both these forms of thinking the significant relation between the mental event (the perceiving or the imagining) and the thing perceived or imagined is that the thing is the principal cause, in a way which we can trace, of the mental event. The thought is of *this* thing rather than *that* because it is *caused* by this thing, not by that. Because it is a *response* to this thing, not to that. A flash of lightning causes in us an experience. How it does so we know in outline. The view which is gaining ground is that this causal connection between the flash and the perceiving of it *is* the knowing relation itself.

Thinking about absent things is essentially reacting as though they were not absent. As Rignano[1] rightly says, thinking is experimentation. It is a process of experimenting not with things, but with their mental representatives. And these representatives are ideas. Ideas will include images as a

---

[1] *The Psychology of Reasoning* (1923). Rignano lays great stress upon *imaginary* experiments; and, with the proviso that actual images need not be involved in them, his account is very clear and helpful.

special sub-class, and also words in some cases. But the majority of the processes in our minds which represent things, and so are ideas, are probably neither images nor words.

Emotional Representation. In certain types, though rarely with those engaged in intellectual activities, the representing idea may be an emotion, a feeling, or a mood. Primitive men, and probably animals, classify and distinguish between objects less by means of representations of them in the strict sense than by revivals of emotions to which they have given rise. These emotive classifications are the germ of all thought, and we tend constantly to fall back upon them, in what, for example, are known as ' intuitive ' judgments of people's personalities. We often judge a new acquaintance to be ' sly ', less from any namable characters of his appearance or behaviour than through the emotion which he arouses. We use the emotion as a sign, overlooking, as far as consciousness goes, the signs which were, of course, necessary for the emotion to arise.

Association. We may now go back to Mr Babbitt and his account, correct so far as it goes, of what we do with our ideas when

we think. First as to how we get them
together. This is what is known as the
association of ideas. The classical doctrine
was that the ruling principle here is contiguity. If two ideas have occurred together
in the past, or if the sources of them, our
contacts with the things which they represent,
were originally together, then the one will
tend to be accompanied again by the other.
This is the obvious consequence of retention
as we studied it in Chapter III, and it
admittedly plays a great part. Other things
being equal, contiguity rules ; but, as later
work has shown, other things seldom are
equal. Contiguity operates only subject to
the guidance of interest. If we are thinking
about niblicks, the ideas which are associated
with the idea of grass will be quite different
from those which will gather if we are thinking about Nebuchadnezzar. The governing
principle in association is the direction of
interest, and contiguity only works inside
this principle. Clearness and consecutiveness
of thinking, in other words, depends primarily
upon clearness in our interests. Perhaps
most of the blunders of thought are due to
confused and mixed interests. The extraordinary views of many demented persons

can be traced to eccentricities of their interests.

We may consider two typical failures in thinking from this point of view, the undue persistence of an irrelevant set of ideas and the failure to hit on the relevant idea even when it ought to be obvious. The first usually springs from an intrusion of interests which have nothing to do with the situation ; the second either from a weakness of the relevant interest or from the same kind of cause as the first. For whatever we may be thinking about on any occasion it is fairly certain that our interests will be far more mixed than we suppose. Now each of our interests acts in a twofold way. It facilitates some processes and inhibits others. And stupidity in the form of overlooking the obvious key-idea of the situation, that distressing but familiar complaint from which we all suffer so constantly, is chiefly a matter of the inhibition of this key-idea by some interest which may be influencing us quite unawares.

Some of the phenomena of forgetting names are illuminating here. We shall understand them better when we have discussed in Chapter XV how the mind goes wrong, but it will be helpful to allude to them now. We often find ourselves forgetting one name out of a group, it may even be the name we are most familiar with among them. This seems inexplicable until perhaps we notice, after looking it up, that a minute or two later we are slightly depressed and going over in our minds irksome thoughts of things not done or of occasions when we made fools of ourselves. Then we may realize that the name is similar in sound to that of a central figure in these disturbing reflections.

These bizarre twists illustrate the very indirect ways in which our interests can interfere with one another. And a great many of our more puzzling stupidities may be put down to this cause. People very commonly refuse to form new ideas rather owing to the discomfort the ideas would produce than through any real intellectual difficulty. But general stupidity, like forgetting, has wider sources. Apart from gross physiological causes—fever, fatigue, and the like—it may come from insufficient experience and familiarity with the right kinds of situation. We handle our ideas of things much as we handle the things themselves, and no one can be expected to work out in

N

thought what is wrong with a car if he has never had much to do with cars.

Concepts. In addition to the thinking that is a recapitulation, as it were, of the concrete handling of things, there is another, a higher order of thinking, abstract or conceptual thinking as it may be called ; and individuals differ in this even more than they do in the simpler kind of thinking.

We saw in the preceding chapter that we can recognize a chair even when it is seen from an unfamiliar angle. There must be a structure in the mind by which it recognizes not this or that particular sensory pattern, but any one of a vast range of patterns which are indifferently taken for the chair. Similarly going a stage higher, we have structures which recognize not this or that chair, but any chair ; and, higher still, a piece of furniture as such. This hierarchy of higher and higher co-ordinating perceptual structures is paralleled in thinking. Our particular *ideas* of individual cars stand to our general idea or 'concept' of a car just as the particular sensory patterns which the chair may present stand to our recognition of it as the chair. The concept is a higher level co-ordinating structure which responds indifferently to any one of an indefinitely large range of particular representations. And it may in abstract thinking operate in conjunction with other concepts without the aid of any *particular* representations at all. When this abstract thinking gets into difficulties we fall back upon particular representations, often in the form of images, in order to see where we are going wrong, just as we look again at the chair if for any reason our first recognition of it seems to be misleading us. We climb down from our higher level, so to speak.

People differ enormously in the level at which they think most successfully and in the degree to which they develop these higher structures and can get ahead without constant recourse to particular representations. Great practical success, as with many business men, engineers, and doctors, is possible without abstract ideas or concepts. For success in the wider understanding of things, however, they are indispensable and they offer innumerable short cuts even in the most practical matters. But, as is well known, short cuts have their dangers, and the theorist who cannot climb down and get back to facts and instances soon becomes a lost man.

The Influence of Language on Thought.
Most abstract thinking tends easily to wander.
Thus a concrete record, plan, or scheme of
its steps is invaluable to it. This it is one
of the main functions of language to provide,
though not, as we have seen (Chapter IX),
its primary or original function. Words
strung together give a kind of mechanical
model of thinking. In the case of mathematics, which by starting from the simplest
aspects of things has become the most
developed form of abstract thinking, the
words, the symbolism, employed to represent
the steps and stages of the thinking have
become nearly perfect. But ordinary language is a comparatively crude representation
of thinking. This is partly because it has
other simultaneous jobs to do as well. It
reflects the thinker's attitudes to things as
well as his thoughts about them, and it is
bent and twisted throughout in the interests
of communication. For language, in addition
to serving the thinker himself, is used in
order to make other people go through the
same thinking processes. The troubles which
this entails are unending. The moral for
all discussion is that we should not mistake
the verbal formulation for the thought itself,

and should remember that it is always at best an imperfect representation of it.[1]

There is another aspect of this influence of language upon thought which should be mentioned. It is often said that we get many of our concepts given us ready-made by language. We should notice that this is only a loose and superficial way of talking. We get the words, but the thoughts in connection with which we use them are our own achievement, helped, of course, immensely by intercourse with others. A very great number of our words and forms of speech we use without any corresponding concepts. We make a purely conventional use of them, uttering them on the same sorts of occasions as other people do, and without thought. But when we do think with them our thinking is the product of our own experience carried up to one level or another ; and thus the thoughts of people using the same words may be, as we are always painfully discovering, very different. It would

[1] For a discussion of these aspects of language see the author's *The Meaning of Meaning*, pp. 358-360 ; also Richards, *Principles of Literary Criticism*, p. 261—further elaborated in his *Practical Criticism* (1929), which may be read in conjunction with Dr June Downey's *Creative Imagination* (1929) for an application of modern psychological principles to the study both of literature in general and of poetry in particular.

be convenient if concepts could be acquired ready-made in this fashion, but actually they have to be arrived at by more arduous means. Educators in particular should never forget that to give the language is one thing and to cause corresponding concepts to be developed is quite another.

Thinking is often described in terms of beliefs, judgments, propositions, assumptions, hypotheses, and arguments.[1] A belief would by many schools be described as a group of ideas united by an act of judgment which predicates some of these ideas of others, thus forming a proposition, which as a whole is asserted. The stringing together of such assertions would constitute argument or discursive thought. This type of analysis is usually encountered in the introductory chapters of treatises on logic. It has a long and distinguished history, since the discussion of the thought processes in a narrow sense and in almost complete separation from the other aspects of mental activity, made up until comparatively recently the major part of psychology. For some of the logician's

---

[1] How psychology may be treated by the very acute thinkers who have favoured the logical and mathematical approaches will be gathered from Professor Moore's *Philosophical Studies*, chap. ii.

special purposes it has its advantages, but it presents an essentially artificial view of thinking. As so often in psychology, the distinctions which are convenient for one purpose are misleading, unless they can be reinterpreted, for another. We have refused throughout these pages to regard ideas, images, or perceptions as entities independent of the activities in the course of which they arise. We must treat judgments, beliefs, propositions and hypotheses in the same way.

It would follow that the difference between a belief or a proposition which is accepted and asserted and one which is merely entertained, supposed, or assumed, is, apart from differences in the belief feelings which we discuss in the next chapter, a difference in the way in which we use them. They are groups of ideas which are formed in the service of our interests. They are ways in which our interests are working themselves out. A settled belief is an arrangement of ideas which in a certain field of occasions is going to be used to control action. Provisional beliefs, hypotheses, and assumptions are arrangements which are being experimented with, on a large or on a small scale. The difference is paralleled exactly in our handling of objects, even in cases where no reflection and no consciousness intervene. We handle liquids and solids, for example, quite differently ; and our most settled beliefs are those which correspond to such routines of daily experience and behaviour.

Any such functional group of ideas as a belief has, of course, an intricate internal structure : these units of thought may take all the forms which experience suggests and, in mathematics, for example, new forms which only prolonged experimentation could have evolved. Many of these patterns of thought are indirectly represented in grammar. Compare 'He will come' with 'He may come'. But grammar is nearly always ambiguous. The difference here may be in the group of ideas itself, a looser structure in the second example ; or it may lie not in the group of ideas, but in our attitude to it as a whole, to 'his coming' as a unit, the same in both cases. To take another pair of examples. Much controversy has raged round the question whether the 'time-element' in 'He fell' and 'He will fall' is in the 'proposition' (i.e., in psychological language, the group of ideas) or in our attitude to it. It is possible to be extraordinarily subtle

over the point in the language of ' propositions'
and ' propositional functions '—the language
of mathematical logic—but it seems unlikely
on general grounds that the mind is incapable
of handling the difference in both ways.
In all such problems of analysis everything
depends, of course, upon our purpose and
the context in which we make the assertion.

The logical analysis of thinking, then, is
neither a rival to nor in conflict with the
psychological, though it may often seem to
be so. Here, as constantly in psychology,
we have to deal with what amounts to a
double or triple staffing of the system—if
we may compare the ideas by which we think
about mental happenings with the personnel
which directs a railway. It would be very
inconvenient to have two or more staffs
looking after the same branch line if their
aims were, as here, divergent, and it seems
reasonable that the special interests and
conceptions of the logicians should give way
to the more general claims of psychology.[1]
They will in the end lose nothing by so
doing.

[1]Such works as *Possibility* (Buchanan, 1927), *The Technique
of Controversy* (Bogoslovsky, 1928), and *The Growth of Reason*
(Lorimer, 1929), give a good idea of the growing tendency
to stress or to adopt the modern psychological approach.

Much light is likely to be thrown on the processes of thought by further study of the various forms of loss of speech (aphasia). Injuries to the brain give rise to very curious disabilities, and the relation of thought to speech has only recently been approached by pathologists with sufficient understanding to take advantage of the opportunities they offer.[1]

We must now turn to consider the emotional side of life. As we have suggested, much of the difficulty and confusion of thinking is only explicable when we take account of this other aspect of our mental activities.

[1] Cf. Piéron, *Principles of Experimental Psychology*, (1929), Part IV, Chapter II.

CHAPTER XIV

EMOTION AND CHARACTER

OUR emotions are the most obscure part of our lives, and, as might be expected, the theory of emotion is the most backward part of psychology. This is the reason for postponing detailed consideration of it to so late a stage, not any minor or secondary importance of the emotional aspect of experience and behaviour. On the contrary, the history of a life is a history of interests rather than of ideas ; and, if we could follow it closely enough, we should find that an understanding of the emotional situation was at every turn the key to the rest. Moreover, it is on his emotional organization that a man's character essentially depends.

Emotional Reverberation. A surprising amount is known already about the phenomena of emotion and the difficulty is less due to a lack of data than to indecision as to what is to be called cause and what effect among these phenomena. Let us examine first the theory around which most recent discussion has revolved.[1] This is the celebrated Lange-James hypothesis of organic resonance, so called after the two adherents who first brought it into prominence.

In fear, the perception of an alarming object, or of an alarming change in the situation, is followed not only by characteristic action, but by an extensive agitation all through the body. Changes take place in the digestive, respiratory, glandular, and circulatory organs. Our hair stands on end, we blush or grow pale, we sweat, our pupils dilate, our digestive canal is paralysed, our pulse quickens, and so forth. Most of these changes are brought about through the agency of the sympathetic nervous system. This is a part of what is known as the 'involuntary' or 'autonomic' nervous system, which looks after our vegetative life and sees to the co-ordinations required in order that our internal organs shall work

[1] An able survey of the whole subject of emotion, with an attempt to arrive at four 'primary' emotions, and an elaborate analysis of 'love' as distinguished from 'sex', will be found in W. M. Marston's *Emotions of Normal People* (1928). It is by the discovery of a scientific basis for a small number of primary emotions that the hitherto mysterious 'analogy' of sound and colour, which has inspired so many artists and baffled so many scientists, may ultimately be explained.

together. It is partially independent of the central or ' voluntary ' nervous system which we discussed in Chapters III-V ; but the degree of this independence is disputed. The supplementary diagram in Figure I shows the relationship between the spinal roots and the sympathetic chain.

The Sympathetic System. The involuntary system is composed of three sections. There is a ' cranial ' section whence a nerve supply is distributed to the heart, lungs, stomach, and intestines, to the arteries of the salivary glands, to the muscles which contract the pupil of the eye and to the tear glands. Parallel to part of the spinal cord there are two chains of ganglia (one of these chains appears in Fig. I) running down parallel with the spinal cord, and distributing a nerve supply to these same organs ; to the liver, spleen, etc. ; to visceral and peripheral arteries ; to the smooth muscles which move the hairs ; to the adrenal glands ; perhaps to the skeletal muscles ; and also to the colon, the bladder, the arteries of the external genitals, and the internal genitals : this nervous organization makes up the ' sympathetic ' system. Thirdly, there is the ' sacral ' section which supplies more directly this last set (colon, etc.). The cranial and sacral sections together are as a rule antagonistic to the sympathetic in their effects ; but the sympathetic usually wins in a struggle between them. The cranial and sacral sections in general promote fairly specific reactions in the organs they serve ; their neurones go directly to ganglia in or near to these organs : but the sympathetic system promotes very diffused and widespread reactions ; the neurones which leave the spinal cord go to ganglia close to it whence diverge other (' post-ganglionic ') fibres in all directions.

One further point should be mentioned to make this sketch sufficiently complete for our purposes. Among the organs supplied by the sympathetic system alone are two small bodies above the kidneys, namely the adrenal glands to which reference was made above. These secrete and discharge into the blood-stream a substance known as adrenalin which, in extraordinarily minute amounts, has, when carried by the blood to organs innervated by the sympathetic, precisely the same effect as if they were receiving nervous impulses from the sympathetic. By this mechanism the power of the sympathetic is enormously increased. But adrenalin produces other effects as well, of which the most important is a facilitation of the supply of fuel to the muscles and a replacement of chemical compounds broken down in muscular work. Thus this liberation of adrenalin through the action of the sympathetic explains both the increased exertion possible in emotional excitement and the reduction of fatigue.

We rarely appreciate the extent and complexity of the autonomic reactions that are constantly occurring in our normal daily life. In sudden emotional shocks, they are fairly evident ; but it is not easy to realize that our internal organic economy undergoes marked variations as our gaze wanders from the clouds to the daisies on the lawn. If the subject be suitably connected with a galvanometer it is found that his resistance varies with changes in his affective condition. This gives us a new and very delicate method of exploring his emotional reactions.[1] The emotional effects of colours and musical notes, so difficult to explain, must probably be traced to these reflex organic resonances.

[1] See Whately Smith, *The Measurement of Emotion* (1922), for a recent discussion of the problems raised by this ' psychogalvanic reflex', based on 45,000 observations.

In fact, as the subtler, less easily described effects of our surroundings upon consciousness show, this ever-present background of organic sensibility (the cenesthesia, as it is called) is one of the most important factors in our lives. It is the basis of our feelings of familiarity and strangeness, and plays a great part in orientating us in all our daily affairs. Violent disturbances of it, due to gross physiological causes, seem to have much to do with some forms of insanity, in which the patient may complain, for example, that he is made of glass or full of frogs, and spend much time endeavouring to explain his strange state by many extravagant suppositions and beliefs. It has been suggested further—for example, by Smith Ely Jelliffe—that electrical, climatic, or other influences may act directly upon the autonomic system, so that it can be regarded as a " receptor and transformer of cosmic energy."[1]

The Disguise of the Organic Response. We can now return to the Lange-James hypothesis. This was that the emotions, at least the coarser of them, were made up of

---

[1] Admirers of Mr D. H. Lawrence's introspective descriptions will be interested in this suggestion. It is also thought by some psychologists that the practices of the Yoga adepts may produce a change in the balance of the autonomic system.

the effects in consciousness of these changes
in the tone of the organs brought about
by the involuntary nervous system, and princi-
pally by the sympathetic. One important
addition is fairly obvious.[1] In an emotion the
organic disturbance is not necessarily recognized for what it is. Or to put it the other
way round, when it is recognized the emotion
is changed and, it may be, dissipated.

Most people have noticed the brusque
transition from an emotion to a neutral
awareness of gooseflesh, trembling, sickness,
breathlessness, and so on, which sometimes
happens. It is a commonplace that we
can show all the signs of fear without actually
experiencing fear, the emotion. We may
note the signs ourselves and say: " How
curious ! I seem to be afraid, but I am not."
A good instance is a sudden ' appalling '
noise which we recognize instantly as nothing
that we need bother about. Shortly afterwards the whole organic reaction ensues,

---

[1] It would be premature to go further on the physiological
side than to point out that the behaviour of certain American
cats, whose sympathetic systems have been removed, is likely
to render the whole subject of the sources of emotion, motor
consciousness, etc., a matter of acute controversy during the
next few years. Recent physiological theory certainly tends
to shew, in opposition to the James-Lange view, that the
cerebral cortex may exercise a controlling function, and that
the true centre of origin of emotional consciousness lies in the
mid-brain.

o

with its leaping pulse, it shivers down the backbone, and the rest of it. But *then* these phenomena appear as what they are and have no tinge of the genuine thrill of fear. Certain bad actors and actresses in particular can cause us violent visceral perturbations, yet we remain *emotionally* quite unmoved.

Projection. A great deal of our experience undergoes, as it occurs, a peculiar and very important transformation. Instead of seeming to be where its neural counterpart is, it appears from the first to be out in the external world whence the stimulus to which it is due originates. Visual objects and ordinary sounds, for example, we irresistibly locate outside us. This process is known as *projection*. But very low or very shrill noises may seem in comparison to be in the ear, and the pain of a pin-prick is very definitely in us, not in the pin. No projection takes place. Intermediate cases occur with perceptions of warmth and cold. Sometimes it is we who are hot, sometimes the sun. An especially interesting case is that of movements. A dizzy man with eyes open sees the world revolving, with eyes shut he himself revolves. Much of our perception of forms, notably of architectural forms, involves projection either of slight movements of our own or of images of such movements. Thus a mountain rises and a steeple soars. Actually we do not doubt that it remains stationary but our projected movements lend it a curious and important appearance of life and movement. This special form of projection is known as Empathy or Einfühlung.

The difference, then, between an emotion and a mere organic disturbance is in part in the degree of projection. Chimpanzees, we saw, when in emotion, tend to do *something*, no matter what, in the direction of the object which has moved them. It is reasonable to take this as a sign of projection. In ourselves, emotions are nearly always projected. We think of the emotion which a picture causes us as a character of it, namely its beauty, much as we assume the perception of red which it may cause in us to be a redness, in some part of it. In the same way we tend, unless very sophisticated, to regard all the objects of our emotions as possessing qualities which, when we look more closely into the matter, we find to be merely projections of our own reactions. Such qualities are nobility, splendour, niceness, ugliness, and rhythm. Sometimes, as in these cases, we have independent names for them. Sometimes we use names which derive from the names of our reactions—pleasant, disgusting, charming, hateful, appalling. In both cases the fact of projection makes an immense difference to our response, not only as an organic reverberation, but in the ways in which we behave towards the object. We have already noted the special prominence of projection in child psychology and in the form of ' eidetic ' phenomena, and in the next Chapter this aspect of the matter will occupy us again.

Incipient Action. Besides the organic discharge, or the representation of it, there is in every emotion another set of effects. The perception which gives rise to the emotion instigates a process of preparation for action. We have only to watch a football crowd to see how at every crisis the spectators more or less unwittingly get ready themselves to do what they hope will be done. And even when we cannot actually observe these preliminary settings of the muscles for action there is reason to suppose that very extensive processes of preparation take place at higher levels. These higher level settings, totally different in the case of fear and rage, for example, seem very largely to make the difference between the emotions ; for they govern our responses and, when we do not go so far as overt action, they are our response. Thus the difference between being frightened and being made merely to quiver may be largely a matter of the extent to which our response develops.

Conflict and Emotion. But here we come across a striking fact which again shows how complex emotional phenomena must be. When our response is complete, instantaneous, and unimpeded, we have no emotional experience at all. We step out of the way of a car without a qualm. When we know what to do and can do it at once we feel nothing. And this is so even when the chances of destruction remain very high. So long as there is something definite to be done we are free from fear. And to a large extent this is so with all the emotions. The lover's agitation takes on a much more moderate tone as soon as he is assured of acceptance. The Corsican bandit is reputed to sight his piece at an enemy with a dispassionate eye, being assured both of escape and of approbation. It seems certain that some degree of conflict between rival tendencies, rival responses to the situation, is required for the full development of emotion.

In cases of pathological forgetting, when a hidden activity seems to be interfering with the main stream, notably by causing groundless emotion, and yet cannot be readily made conscious, the unconscious activity is said to be *repressed*. We shall discuss repression in the following chapter. Here we need only note that the repressing agent is probably the successful activity itself ; though it is not necessarily aware that it is repressing anything. A ' forbidden ' activity which, if it were successful, would cause a predominantly pleasant emotion, may, when defeated, lead to an emotion of anxiety. It is as though the danger which it offers to the triumphant activities were the source of the emotion. And in fact these activities are, in the measure in which the repressed tendency is strong, in a state of insecurity. We may often misinterpret this sense of anxiety, supposing, for example, that it is due to the dangers of modern traffic when actually it springs from the partial success of Potiphar's wife.

The causes of our emotions are, it follows, not always so obvious as they often appear.

It is a commonplace that joys spring from the temporary rout of distresses, and there is reason to suppose that this is true in a deeper sense. For the normal condition of the mind is one of strain, a great number of tendencies being with difficulty repressed. The characteristic condition of elation is one in which either a very complete momentary triumph of some group of impulses has taken place—possibly after a sudden resolve which may lead either to a conversion or to a debauch—or in which there has been a re-organization of the mind which gives hitherto repressed tendencies a new means of co-operating with their former opponents. In the one case a swing of the pendulum is taking place ; in the other the pendulum has been rehung.

Belief and Doubt. It remains to discuss two other topics which less evidently come under the heading of emotional phenomena. One of these includes belief, doubt, prejudice, and so forth ; the other, deliberation, resolve, and the fluctuations of the will. As experiences all these are essentially emotional. We often say that a man holds such and such beliefs, is sceptical in such and such matters, or that he is bigoted, determined, irresolute, or changeable, when we do not thereby intend to describe his experience, but merely to indicate his typical ways of behaving. In these cases we are referring to the more or less permanent dispositions which determine what he will do, and these dispositions may operate without any awareness on his part. Many beliefs in this sense are formed without any feeling accompaniment.

As dispositions our beliefs are unconscious, and since they may operate without our awareness we find that many doubts and decisions are also unconscious. But when we analyse the states of consciousness known by these names we find that the distinctive character of a crisis of belief or doubt is a feeling, of the same general kind as joy, for example, or fear, though unique in flavour. Expectation, bare assent, and familiarity are examples of such belief feelings. They are generally less intense than emotions, although pathological forms of doubt and ecstatic belief are not infrequent. Both seem able to occur in cases where there is nothing definite which is either doubted or believed. In the nitrous oxide and mescal exaltations, for example, anything can be believed to a degree of intensity which quite overshadows waking conviction [1] ; and in doubting manias everything can be doubted. The patient may sometimes even doubt whether he exists.

It may be added that the intensity of the belief-feeling is no criterion of the permanence of the disposition which it leaves behind. Many people who experience the most intense beliefs are also the most changeable and instable in their convictions. As a rule in such cases and in normal life, the belief or doubt feelings are very subtly interwoven with the other emotions. We rarely believe strongly unless some emotion—it may be joy or fear, pride or humility—is reinforcing the belief. And doubt, more evidently, perhaps, is commonly dependent upon a prior clash of interests and a resultant emotion.

But if these intellectual feelings spring from other emotions they also give rise to them, since they modify so fundamentally the course of our responses. Strong belief is almost always the sign of the triumph of

[1] Cf. Leuba, *The Psychology of Religious Mysticism* (1925), pp. 27, 274-275. Leuba's work was the first to render accessible the material for a comparison of the emotional states produced by the various drugs with those in which a religious element predominates. A strangely neglected field of investigation is opened up here ; and H. Klüver's *Mescal* (1928) has since added considerably to our knowledge of the action of this ' divine plant ' of the American Indians.

some important interest. It may be a grounded triumph in the case of a Galileo and his pendulum, or an ungrounded triumph as with an inebriate and his lamp-post. Even scepticism is for many people a source of infinite ironic delight.

Deliberation and Resolve. The experiences of deliberation and resolve are plainly very similar to beliefs and doubts. Doubt is a special form of irresolution. We may, it is true, ' make up our minds ' and form a resolve without any definite belief, either that we are following the best course or that the situation requires it ; but supporting beliefs very commonly develop. And such beliefs, when they are due to our being already involved in a line of action with a certain amount of our energy and time invested in it, rather than to evidence, are typical prejudices. As we shall see in the next chapter, the majority of our prejudices are unconscious ; whence the notorious difficulty of proving to anyone that he is prejudiced.

The Sentiments. The majority of adult emotions arise only in connection with what are known technically as the sentiments. A sentiment is a group of interests organized around a set of objects or ideas. Typical instances are friendships, antipathies, the self-regarding sentiment, and the sentiment of patriotism. Sometimes a conflict between sentiments, common in childhood, may occur. Then, if the rivalry cannot be solved by a reorganization of one or other or both of them, a whole group of interests may be repressed. Such repressed sentiments, and sentiments which in general are out of accord with the main body of sentiments which makes up the character, are known as *complexes*. With these we shall be more concerned in the following Chapter.

CHAPTER XV

HOW THE MIND GOES WRONG

Character and the Unconscious. By a man's 'character' at any time we may mean either his dominant sentiments and beliefs or the whole system of all his sentiments and complexes, conscious and unconscious alike, the entire organization of his dispositions. This last is perhaps better named his personality.[1] Psycho-analysts have rather overworked their explanations, which, although developed chiefly in connection with morbid conditions of mind, have succeeded none the less in revealing a great deal about human nature of which good self-observers were already aware. " Forgetfulness ", wrote

[1] A discussion which brings out the physiological and psychical bases of character particularly well will be found in *Personality,* by Dr R. G. Gordon (1926). It contains also one of the least biased accounts of the varieties of psycho-analytic theory which have yet appeared, and is supplemented by the same author's *The Neurotic Personality* (1927). Dr A. A. Roback's *The Psychology of Character* (1925) is a notable example of the voluminous literature motivated by current educational or moral interests.

Nietzsche in 1886, " is no mere *vis inertiæ*, as the superficial believe ; rather is it a power of obstruction, active, and, in the strictest sense of the word, positive . . . a very sentinel and nurse of psychic order, repose, and etiquette."[1]

Six years later appeared the first works of Freud in which the theory of repression and transformation was given definite shape. Forel in 1874 had proved the suppression and transformation of instincts in ants, but Freud contended that the suppressed instinct may discharge itself in other forms, and may continue to exhibit itself either in a ' neurosis ' or in a ' sublimation '—*i.e.*, a socially approved form of activity.

The Mutual Obstruction of Interests. Colloquially we say of a man suffering from a mental disorder that ' he is all tied up in knots inside ', and this comparison does faithfully represent what in fact has happened. Psycho-analysis, in fact, is essentially a ' jam-probe '.[2] His interests (and we must remember that an interest is an activity springing from a need) instead of allowing smooth

---

[1] Cf. Prof. C. Baudouin, " The Evolution of Instinct from the Standpoint of Psycho-analysis," *Psyche*, vol. iii, 1922, p. 5.

[2] A useful American term for ' an inquiry into traffic congestion.'

and clear passage to one another are in some way mutually obstructive. The working of one is hindering that of others and, it may be, involving activity which has nothing to do with the situation and is out of place.

We saw, in describing how the child's mind grows, that it begins as a system of interests which are very unlike those with which it concludes as a healthy adult. We saw that the infant's view of the world is a reflection of his interests, and the adult's a reflection of his. The immense difference in their world pictures corresponds to an equal difference in their interests. Now the most extensive and the most abrupt of the changes in interest occur in early years. Hence the stress which Freud has rightly laid upon infantile experience as a determining cause of later mental life. And further, the most important of the child's interests, and of the adult's, are those which make up the system governing his relations to other human beings. And since he grows up from complete dependence to partial freedom, all the while in peculiarly close contact with his parents, there is nothing surprising in the view that the kind of interest he takes in them and the way this interest changes will greatly influence his later life. **The Freudian Theory of Sex.** What was surprising and gave the world in general a beneficial shock was Freud's persistence in regarding these interests as sexual. The Freudians have been led largely through the study of certain eccentricities in adults to point to particular infantile situations as origins of special sub-trends in later life. For example the infant's acts of evacuation, which, as all mothers know, assume great importance in his sight, may, through their special sexual interest, later influence his attitudes to gifts and to money. This is the Freudian explanation of the miser's love of gold.[1] And the same kind of stage-to-stage *transference* (a fundamental conception in psycho-analysis as indeed in all psychology, since it is only substitution or conditioning seen from another angle) would extend the infant's original love of touching

[1] There are, of course, many steps and turnings in such a transference. A lucid account of the child's growth will be found in J. H. van der Hoop, *Character and the Unconscious*, Ch. iii. Dr Nathan Miller's *The Child in Primitive Society* (1928) is a mine of information for all who are concerned with the protection of the young from the psychological horrors of the past ; and may be read in conjunction with Professor Bronislaw Malinowski's instructive *Sex and Repression in Savage Society* (1927), where exception is taken to certain of Freud's generalizations, or with Dr Otto Rank's *The Trauma of Birth* (1929), which elaborates one of his more speculative suggestions.

and being touched (handling and being handled) into the delight so many find in ordering their lovers about (sublimated sadism) or being ordered about by them (sublimated masochism.) Similarly with the child's passion for displaying himself and for looking at others. There is a sense in which the pervert is one who has *remained* rather than *become* such, and may be regarded as exhibiting a form of inhibited development.

The Riddle of the Sphinx. The most important of all cases of transference concerns the parents. The mother's (or nurse's) predominance does not, of course, last for long. The father and any brothers and sisters there may be come into the picture, and the job of reconciling and adjusting the multitude of different interests which arise becomes very complex. As was noted in Chapter VIII, the child easily regards both what happens in him as happening outside him (Projection, as the analysts call it) and what happens outside as happening in him (Introjection). The boundaries of his self are not yet established. His thoughts of his father and mother are not and cannot yet be clearly marked off for him from his father and mother themselves, and his interest in them is

predominantly selfish. But at the same time
their behaviour and the differences between
them give him all the patterns for his own
activities, and in working out these patterns
he both projects and introjects continually.
He sees himself in them and he finds them
in himself. There is nothing in the least
surprising, then, if we find him, as we do,
constantly behaving to his father as his
mother does and to his mother as his father.

The Œdipus complex is the name for a
particular system of these activities. Œdipus
in the legend, after guessing the riddle of
the Sphinx, became a king and married the
reigning queen who in fact was his mother.
Freud believes that in the phantasies of
every child (or rather in the wish-activities
from which phantasies spring) this drama is
re-enacted. There comes a point when a
boy wishes to replace his father in his mother's
affections, and a girl wishes to replace her
mother. And Freud holds (which is the point
at which opposition chiefly arises) that this
wish may be very specific and definite. It
varies in many ways, but chiefly with the
degree to which the riddle of the Sphinx
has been guessed.

This riddle is nothing else than the great

P

problem, for the child, as to how he came to be born. This problem and its clue, the difference between the sexes, inevitably exercise every child enormously. There *may* be something to be said for keeping him ignorant once the desire for knowledge has been expressed, on the ground that it gives him his first real training in scientific research, but these advantages are far outweighed by the distortions of his personality produced in an atmosphere of secrecy. That he should appear to drop the subject may be convenient for bashful parents, but is really a bad sign. He should—and this is one of the most important practical recommendations that it is possible for psychology to give—have his problem well ventilated for him and be given, not hurriedly as something unpleasant to be got over, but freely and without poetic nonsense, all the data which he needs.

The child's crude theories (and no child is without them) of the differences between the sexes are particularly important. The boy, briefly, is proud of his possessions, and the girl rather resentful of what she regards as an unfair deficiency. By very natural analogies the boy may come to dread that he will some day suddenly be turned into a girl. This dread, and the resultant theories and phantasies to which it leads, is known as the castration complex. It may afterwards have startling consequences if he becomes predominantly attached to his father. Certain threats sometimes used to children may favour this dread. In the girl whose psychology is very much more obscure, for as yet there has been no feminine Freud, a different complex may develop, though one equally capable of playing a part in after life—an infantile sense of unfair treatment which may greatly strengthen all the other better grounded reasons which women may later have for a quarrel with the natural order of things. The castration complex, for the girl, appears as a notion or fear that she is but an imperfect man.

Conflict and Repression. We come now to the problem of the interaction of all these queer interests as they become more specific. The life of a healthy child from birth until towards five years old may be regarded as a time of more or less independent development of its manifold sexual and other interests. But by growing severally more definite they are obviously heading for a time when they will interfere with one another. One of the chief clashes comes, according to Freud, at about five years over the Œdipus complex. We must not suppose that the boy (*vice versa* if a girl) is then merely in love with his mother and anxious only that his father shall be dead (= vanished). At the same time he may be passionately attached to his father. And out of this contradiction trouble may arise.

One common form of temporary solution is the *repression* of the interest either in the mother or in the father. This notion is fundamental; it is also the point at which metaphors usually begin to become misleading. Repression we have insisted is simply inhibition, the universal phenomenon we considered in Chapter III. A repressed wish is a set of impulses cut off temporarily or permanently from the final common paths.

It may happen that whereas impulses from the whole up-to-date co-ordinated need cannot get through, impulses from the component needs can ; then through a backwash influence the need reverts to an earlier stage of development, and we have what is known as *regression*. The child's comparatively developed sexual interest is transformed to an earlier type. To a type, for instance, for which the difference between the sexes is no longer significant, it returns suddenly from a four-year-old stage to a one-year-old.

Regression. This kind of catastrophe, for such it may be, involves both a lapse backwards of behaviour and a reformation of ideas. For here, as always, the child's understanding and its wishes are different aspects of the same thing. But since not its whole mind, but only one out of its interests, has lapsed back, the common result is a widespread disorder, for some of its ideas which have been developed in the interests of its now lapsed interest are also involved in other interests which have not lapsed. Thus further conflicts arise. Partial and permanent regression, in other words, is a bad solution. Brief *temporary* regressions may, on the other hand, be very useful. The parent who can make them in his play with children is a great success.

Mechanisms of the Unconscious. A repressed wish is usually described as being forced into the Unconscious, and it is often supposed to be active there in the same way as before, much as a submarine continues as before when it dips below the surface. And between the Unconscious and the Conscious another department of the mind is supposed to intervene, namely the Fore- or Pre-conscious, which in complicated ways helps to rule the relations between these domains. It must be realized that these divisions are merely conveniences introduced in order to make exposition more easy. As soon as we forget this they become inconveniences, in fact such a scheme is far too simple, and the real interactions of different interests are far too subtle to be described so simply. It is true that a repressed wish is not thereby abolished, yet we should not suppose it to continue unchanged by repression. What makes it appear to be unchanged is the fact that, later on, behaviour may appear which is unmistakably activated by an exactly similar wish. This, of course, is no proof of an underground persistence of the wish itself, any more than the return of Spring each year is a proof that she has been lurking in the soil throughout the winter. What persists in all cases is a certain pattern in the organization of the mind. If the need behind the wish persists and conditions once again allow this pattern to be used, the wish reappears all complete. But that is a very different thing from its having itself been striving for manifestation throughout the interval. For example, given strawberries, I may at once wish for cream, but this does not mean that a wish for cream has been battering for months at the barred gates of consciousness and has now seized its chance. The point, as we can easily see, is that the specific need for cream only arose with the coming of the strawberries. But with many wishes that, unlike the wish for cream, unfortunately cannot be expressed, the equivalent of the strawberries is always coming. They are always being touched off either by cyclically recurrent organic states, or by patterns in the external stimulation which may be very hard to separate out and distinguish. And since other simultaneous needs and their resultant wishes are in possession of the appropriate final common paths, the wishes these needs give rise to can only find satisfaction either by reorganizing their needs backwards or forwards (regression or development) or by some kind of compromise with their rivals at the gateways to action. It is these compromises which give rise to many of the phenomena of dreams, and in more serious cases to those disorders of the mind which are known as *neuroses,* as well as to innumerable more trifling oddities and mistakes in ordinary life.

Compromises. Such compromises between conscious wishes which interfere with one another are familiar to everyone. A man wishes to take a holiday and also to get on with his work. If he can he takes his work with him and so combines the two. But conscious wishes are only those which are not in too direct conflict with the main systems which the individual is prepared to avow freely and has recognized as belonging to him. Certain sets of wishes he constantly hears acknowledged by his friends; his mechanisms of projection and introjection lead him readily to recognize these in himself. Some he will find acknowledged only in the best fiction; to these he will give a more private kind of recognition. But a swarm of others long ago came into direct conflict either with the wishes of parents and elders or with other avowed wishes of his own. These wishes are not conscious, and he may easily be quite unable to believe that he has them if to avow them would in any way upset his self-esteem; and this very early begins to turn upon the character of his avowed wishes, since to avow some wishes, but not others, is usually the highway to parental esteem.

In his more recent work (especially *Beyond the Pleasure Principle*) Freud has developed from this branch of his theory a threefold division of the psyche, into the Id (German, *das Es*), the Ego, and the Ego-ideal or super-Ego. The Id is the original elementary unconscious psychic mass out of which the personality is differentiated and grows. Impulses in the Id follow the *pleasure principle* ; they satisfy themselves at all costs—with actualities if possible, but otherwise with phantasies and day-dreams. In time, however, the child is forced by experience to face facts and comes under the *reality-principle*, recognizing that the facts conflict with his satisfactions. Out of this recognition grows the Ego—a part of the Id modified by the influence of the outer world. It is an elaborate system, partly conscious and partly unconscious, partly in conflict with the Id and partly ready to find means to indulge the Id. Out of this division, again, grows the super-Ego, a critical portion of the Ego that tries to impose the wishes of the parents, or of society, or of moral heroes with which the child has in the past *identified* himself, upon the Ego and the Id. This influence of the super-Ego is what our ancestors christened ' conscience '. But since it derives from these identifications (which are themselves a form of gratification, under the pleasure-principle rather than the reality-principle) the super-Ego is, in a sense, nearer than the Ego to the Id. Hence, the blind, ' transcendental ', and sometimes ' irrational ' tendency displayed by Conscience, and its frequent incapacity to accept compromises or take account of what is possible and prudent.[1]

Dream Analysis. In the dream, or rather in one very frequent type of dream, we have a figurative sketch of the solution of a conflict ; usually this is an absurd solution, though sometimes, as some notable scientific discoveries show, it may have value. Sleep has cut off the greater part of stimulation, and it has altered the whole scheme of

---

[1] An excellent summary and discussion of Freud's later views on this matter will be found in *Problems of Psychopathology* (1928), by T. W. Mitchell, M.D., where the situation which gives rise to various derangements of the mind is described as follows :—" We thus get a picture of the Ego assailed on three sides, in bondage to three different masters, each of whom it must satisfy if it is to be free from anxiety. Danger to the Ego may come from the outside world, from the libido of the Id, or from the severity of the Ego-ideal ".

waking inhibitions. Unconscious wishes aroused during the day then find an opportunity for displaying themselves. But conscious wishes, though greatly weakened, are also still active. The dream is a compromise in which none of the wishes operating may be clearly revealed. It may be interpreted, as a rule, in many fashions, corresponding to the wishes involved. As everyone knows, it tends to be very rapidly forgotten ; the conscious wishes reinforced by the waking situation soon make the recall of the compromise impossible. There is nothing particularly mysterious in this. We can cross a stream in a drought which is hopeless in normal weather, and there is no need to suppose any Censor who takes a partial nap with us and is caught off his guard in the dream, or baffled by the disguises of the unconscious. All this is mythological machinery for convenience of exposition. The dream is the product of a transaction between conscious and unconscious wishes and the results during sleep are naturally very different from those during waking hours.

The analysis of the dream consists mainly of allowing ' free associations ', as they are called, to come into the mind in connection with as many as possible of the recalled episodes and features of the dream. These associations are again compromises between conscious and unconscious wishes. They often show what seems an astounding power of recondite metaphorical allusion on the part of the unconscious wish, as any study of dream analysis will show. But the most interesting feature of such dream analyses is the frequency with which infantile wishes reproducing infantile experiences enter into them. One reason for this is fairly clear and helps to explain why dreams occur at all. Being asleep in bed is one of the few among our activities (if we may call it such) which have continued unchanged since infancy. But there are deeper reasons. Most of the wishes which we consciously discountenance were first outlawed in our childish days. They are new productions of the old needs which had such a stormy history long ago, the needs themselves being reinstated by recent situations—generally bearing a subtle resemblance to our old emotional situations. Hence the great importance of the earlier handling of these situations in childhood.

Transference. This reawakening of an old need by a situation which may have only a remote, or trivial, or purely schematic resemblance to the ancient problem is the work of that transference which we have already considered. It is through transference that all our triumphs come—and also most of our woes. Any and every metaphor, simile, or analogy illustrates it. But whereas analogies and most similes usually bring out clearly the relevant point through which the transference is effected, metaphor—poetic metaphor especially—often leaves this point very obscure. So it is with the points of resemblance through which infantile needs are reawakened in later life. For the child's original classifications were very different from the adult's, and his ways of thinking far less systematic than our own. Hence also the apparent incoherence of such dreams.

The infantile need thus awakened, events tend to take the course originally taken. For example, a child for whom the Œdipus situation led to a clash between his love for his mother and his different love for his father may, when he grows up, have his infantile mother-love reawakened by some chance similarity to her in his wife—as judged, of course, by infantile standards. The effect of this will vary with the outcome of the original clash. In fact, a man's outlook on the world and his attitude to other people, especially women, is largely determined by the manner in which the transference from the parents to the outside world, at school or in the ball-room, has been effected.

Such in outline is the modern theory of the ways in which the mind goes wrong. The whole theory is in many quarters rejected. But its opponents sometimes show either ignorance and misconceptions of it or an emotional attitude towards it which suggest that their theoretical objections are in part *rationalizations*, to use a term which we shall explain in the following Chapter.

A number of cleavages have occurred within the ranks of psycho-analysts, and these schisms have led to much unnecessary acrimony. The three main schools—of Freud, of Adler, and of Jung—tend too much to regard their accounts as incompatible. But just as there may be for a dream a number of different but equally good interpretations, so it is with all psychical products and phenomena. We are not yet within several centuries of a complete account, and meanwhile any clue which in any way helps to unravel the maze should be followed up.

Organ-inferiority. Adler's distinctive treatment sets out not from the sexual interests, but from what Freud regards as the other main group—the Ego interests. These other interests, built up round the child's desire for power and reflecting themselves in his ambitions, undergo a process of development corresponding in broad outlines to the processes we have sketched. For Adler the key to character lies in the association of what he has named 'organ-inferiority' with a 'superiority' aim (ambition). A defect of which the child is sensible leads him to an effort at compensation, sometimes successful—as in the case of Napoleon, who complained later that he always felt like 'a boiled fowl' at home, where he was bullied by the family. But sometimes the compensation, the desire to obtain power in other ways, may be disastrous. The typical instance is that of the 'malade imaginaire', who, failing to make himself or herself felt in ordinary life, contrives to turn the rest of the family into a nursing staff. The instance brings out the important point that there is no hard and fast line to be drawn between malingering and mental illness. As Crookshank writes, " Where there is a will not to do, there is always a way of escape from doing what should be done".[1] Most people have plenty of weak spots physically and plenty of awkward problems of mental adjustment, and the tendency to dodge the latter by stressing the former provides a large part of every medical practice.

Moral Re-education. This insistence upon the present problem, as opposed to Freud's insistence upon infantile problems, is in a large measure Jung's contribution to psycho-analytic theory. His famous theory of Types and his doctrine of the Collective Unconscious give rise rather to speculation than to positive results. Jung sees in many, indeed, in most, mental disorders what amounts to a moral failure to meet the exigencies of life, which should be set right, mainly by a re-education of the individual which aims at making him realize his duties and his work in the

---

[1] *Migraine and Other Common Neuroses* (1925), p. 37. A pathetic study of cases on the borderlands of the criminal and the pathological will be found in *Emotion and Delinquency* (1928), by Dr L. Grimberg ; while in Blondel's *The Troubled Conscience* one of the easiest roads to the asylum can be discovered from the language of those who have traversed it to the end.

world. He is thus much more in line with traditional views of the function of the spiritual adviser than the other psychoanalysts, who, however, are by no means blind to this factor in the situation. They reply that most people are only too well aware of what they ought to do and that the real problem is to discover why they cannot do it. On the other hand, by pointing out that failure to reach a *decision*, with its corollary, a Troubled Conscience, may be the unsuspected cause of ailments regarded as obstacles to such a decision, candid friends can and do often set the pilgrim on the right track—back, it may be, to his own fireside.

CHAPTER XVI

THE ABNORMAL

The Borderland. Around the frontiers
of the better established part of psychology
lies a ring of debatable matters ; sometimes
these are treated as though they must involve
quite new hypotheses and principles of explanation ; sometimes an attempt is made
to extend the hypotheses already in use so
as to include them. There are many who
hold that these borderline phenomena—
suggestion, hypnotism, telepathy, clairvoyance, and mediumistic happenings in general
—will involve in the end a reconquest, as
it were, of ordinary psychology by some
form of Animism. The hypotheses needed
to explain, for example, how a mind can act
upon a distant mind (if it does) will, it is
held, when they have been worked out, make
ordinary orthodox psychology seem unduly
timid.

Unfortunately these exceptional phenomena
which lie outside normal psychology are

notoriously hard to observe. They inevitably remain too often at the stage of the remarkable anecdote. Full verification and corroboration are rarely possible. A quite special criticism is required before they can be accepted as fact ; and, in face of the great reserves which their extraordinary nature demands, and the difficulties as regards testimony and even mere accurate description, it is hardly surprising that so much hesitation should be felt by psychologists in admitting them as facts at all. We shall see that different classes of these phenomena stand in different positions in this respect. And such a preliminary sorting out is almost all that psychology can at present do with them.

Suggestion. We may conveniently begin with suggestion, since, although the more striking instances of suggestion are unquestionably abnormal, and in many cases not above suspicion as having been misdescribed and exaggerated, suggestion itself is a quite normal process which can be observed easily enough in ordinary daily life.

In its widest sense ' suggestion ' is merely another name for the working of mental processes in general. A stimulus would 'suggest' its response, and this, whether the stimulus be a perception, an idea, or an emotion, and whether the response be a movement, another idea, or a further emotion. In this sense the sight of a theatre-bill 'suggests' a visit to the play, or a despondent mood 'suggests' a series of melancholy reflections. But the sense of 'suggestion' prominent in recent discussion, for example in the agitation centering round the work of Liébault, of Bernheim, and of Coué, is narrower than this. Only those suggestions which take place primarily through the operation of unconscious processes are included in the narrower sense. Going to the play or indulgence in gloomy prognostications is ordinarily under our own conscious control. They are *voluntary* activities, matters of the will; but sometimes we may find ourselves stepping through the theatre doors when we have strong reasons for being elsewhere or we may harrow ourselves with thoughts which are the last we consciously wish to entertain. Such impulsions or obsessions are typical examples of the working of suggestion in this narrower sense.

The most interesting field for suggestion is in the control of the bodily functions.

As all who suffer from colds are only too well aware, we have very little conscious power of control over what takes place in the nasal passages. But, as the phenomena of faith-healing also show, unconscious control may be very much wider. Not only functional disorders, but some organic conditions also can be corrected by psychological means.[1] Warts, for example, it is said, can be cured in many cases with great ease by the recitation of an appropriate verbal formula.

But the question arises, why are some suggestions effective and others not? The answer given by Coué and his followers at Nancy is that failure is due to the arousal of a counter-suggestion. They draw a very hard and fast line between the ' Will ' and the ' Imagination ', using these terms in their popular sense. It will repay us to examine more closely the distinction. The ' will ' on this view would appear to be the conscious operation of a particular interest or set of interests, whereas the ' imagination '—that

[1] The antithesis between ' organic ' and ' functional ' diseases has, indeed, been abandoned of recent years by medical men who are familiar with the findings of modern psychopathology. In the most unexpected branches of medicine the psychological factor has been found to have a far-reaching influence, as can be seen, for example, from Dr W. J. O'Donovan's *Dermatological Neuroses* (1927), where its close relation to skin diseases is for the first time adequately emphasized.

is, the picturing or thinking of the end to be reached—allows a variety of unconscious wishes to take effect, and gives less occasion for conflicting wishes to interfere. A consciously formulated wish often seems to act as a challenge to any dissentients there may be in the personality, though in many cases, of course, such a wish is quite effective, a point which M. Coué did not sufficiently stress. It all depends upon the strength of the wish and the extent to which it is in conflict with other wishes, or, as Coué put it, with the imagination : " When the will and the imagination are at war, the imagination *invariably* gains the day. In the conflict between the will and the imagination the force of the imagination is *in direct ratio to the square of the will* ". This metaphorical statement becomes more plausible when we realize that the " force of the imagination " is the force of the desires and interests to which the imagining is due. We must, of course, be careful in the examples we choose. M. Coué's favourite instance, the undesirability of *trying*, of making an effort, to go to sleep is clearly misleading, sleep being by the nature of the case a state in which effort must be absent. But when, as for example in getting up on a winter's morning, effort is not antagonistic to the desire to seat oneself at the breakfast table, or even perhaps to reach the office before ten o'clock, the exercise of the will is salutary and successful almost daily ; and this no matter how powerfully the imagination pictures the rigours of the frore morning air.

Auto-suggestion. The controversy as to whether all suggestion is really auto-suggestion —*i.e.*, whether all suggestion involves the intervention of our own imagination, or whether all auto-suggestion ultimately depends on suggestion from without—would seem to be due to a common failure in systematizers to allow for the many ways in which the mind works.

There is no doubt that suggestions of external origin gain added force when they ally themselves with auto-suggestions, and conversely an auto-suggestion will be the stronger if some authoritative utterance from a person of prestige—a doctor, a teacher, or a public idol—is co-operating. None the less these two processes may be regarded as distinct, though, of course, an external suggestion which elicits the support of no conscious or unconscious interest will lead to no response ; whether this interest be an impulse to conform, or to obey—and Binet reduced all suggestion to obedience— to please the suggestor, or to be a satisfactory platform exhibit. The reason for distinguishing between them is that the motives operating in the two cases are usually diverse ; with external suggestion they are largely of social origin.

Hypnosis. This brings us to the problem of the influence of mind upon mind and the vexed question of hypnosis. About 1880 hypnotism emerged suddenly, with the work of Richet and Charcot, from the period of opprobrium which followed the excesses of Mesmer.[1] For a while the most remarkable phenomena were recorded, including the transference of affections from one side of the body to another by means of magnets, anæsthesia, clairvoyance, etc., all leading to the conclusion that the mind could be influenced from without by unknown forms of vibration and radiation. But with the triumph of the Nancy School, which already in the eighties attributed everything to ' suggestion ', though without at that date giving any

---

[1] An absorbing account of the history of animal magnetism and hypnotism will be found in the two volumes of Janet's *Psychological Healing* (1925).

account of it, interest in hypnosis declined. It has generally been supposed that the hypnotizer works upon his subject by restricting the range of his attention, and that this narrowed field of concentrated attention allows the suggestion a free field for operation ; while Freud has recently pointed out that fascination and infatuation, the extreme developments of being ' in love ', are but little removed from hypnosis. The effects of Rhythm in poetry, music, and the arts might also be brought under this heading.

The most characteristic phenomenon of hypnosis, as its name implies, is the inducement of artificial sleep. Sir Michael Foster recorded a case where a man had no sense organ left save a single eye. He was half-blind, totally deaf, and insensible to all other stimuli. If anyone closed his remaining eye he promptly fell asleep. The cutting off of the sole remaining field of attention left him no alternative.

There are signs of a reaction against the view that hypnosis is only a phenomenon of suggestion. It was maintained by the late Dr Alrutz on the basis of a number of ingenious experiments that passes, which used to be so prominent in the procedure of mesmerists and the early hypnotizers, do in fact play an essential part. After covering the subject's head completely with a black cloth, and shielding his arm from currents of air, etc., by sheets of glass, he claimed to have induced by a few downward passes complete insensibility of the skin. Upward passes produced the opposite effect. Precautions against suggestion seem to have been taken.[1]

Whatever may be the truth with regard to these contentions, some of the better established phenomena of the hypnotic state are so extraordinary that the slight amount of work which is being done upon them is surprising. Even major operations—the removal of a leg, for example—were performed without pain before the discovery of anæsthetics, though it has been held that these were less phenomena of hypnosis than of hysteria. It seems possible indeed that had the discovery of chemical anæsthetics been delayed a considerable development in the practical use of hypnosis would have taken place.

Hyperaesthesia. Another well-authenticated phenomenon is what is known as *hyperæsthesia*. The subject in light hypnosis quite usually displays powers of sensory

---

[1] *Psyche*, vol. iv, October, 1923 ; p. 129, ff.

discrimination much superior to those possible in the waking state. Instances are reported in which he is able to perceive distinctly the details in microscopic slides, and to overhear conversations in remote rooms which would normally be inaudible, facts which would seem to show that we do not usually exploit our powers of perception to the full. Doubtless, this hyperaesthesia has a bearing upon many alleged instances of telepathy. In this connection we may recall the controversy, still *sub judice*, between M. Jules Romains and the Sorbonne professors on the subject of ' eyeless sight '. M. Romains claims to have discovered a power of reading through the skin, for which he gives an anatomical and evolutionary explanation, and which may be revived in a suitable " régime of consciousness "—possibly a form of mild hypnosis. Whether or not the facts are as described—and the late Anatole France was among those who vouched for some of them—the problems raised by the discussions are of unusual theoretical interest, and should certainly be further examined.[1]

[1] *Eyeless Sight*, 1923. In his *Social World of the Ants* (2 vols., 1928), Forel gives examples of insect sight which have a bearing on the controversy, without, however, committing himself on either side.

Post-hypnotic Suggestion. If during hypnosis it is suggested to the subject that at a fixed time after waking he shall perform some unusual act, for example remove his shoes and place them in the book-case, he will often perform the act at the appropriate moment—showing incidentally a remarkably accurate appreciation of the lapse of time. When asked why he has done this he will usually give some more or less plausible and elaborate answer, bearing no relation to the real reason, known only to the experimenter. Such answers, known as rationalizations, throw a curious light upon the normal working of the mind, particularly in the matter of political opinion.

Telepathy. The evidence for the influence of mind upon mind independently of the recognized channels of sense has long been accepted by a sufficient number of trustworthy investigators to justify the scientific study which is now being devoted to it. The fact that such trained thinkers as Sidgwick, James, Forel, Freud, Driesch, Bergson, McDougall, Becher, and Broad, to name only a few of those who have actually written on the subject, are convinced of its occurrence, makes the cavalier dismissal of its possibility no longer prudent. We know too little about the nervous system to be sure that an event in one body may not produce a direct effect in another, even at a remote distance. No useful conjectures can yet be made as to how it should do so ; but there certainly seems no reason to assert, for example, that special receptive organs would be required. The absence of such organs, then, is no good ground for a hasty return to the primitive hypothesis, the view, namely, that on exceptional occasions the soul, or a part of it is able to leave the body and travel to distant regions. Nor is an acceptance of telepathy necessarily a step towards Animism. The aim of science is to give an intelligible account of what happens, and to speak in this connection of direct interactions between souls which transcend space or operate in supernumerary dimensions is not, unless something much more definite can be added, particularly profitable. Such accounts, although they may provide a certain emotional satisfaction, actually bring us at present no nearer an understanding of the alleged phenomena. This is in fact a field in which a resort to words which have no definite significance is fatally easy.

Various other phenomena, for which the evidence is less satisfactory, are allied to telepathy and raise similar fundamental issues if they are accepted. Such are clairvoyance and the prediction of the future. In the typical case of clairvoyance the subject, sometimes in a trance-condition, sometimes in what appears to be a quite normal state, reads the contents of an opaque envelope which has been sealed with all possible precautions, or, as in the celebrated ' book tests ', indicates the words or matter of a passage of print in some volume which has been set aside with others for the purposes of the experiment in a distant house, after the most elaborate precautions have been taken to prevent any collusion. In this last instance it would appear that no one whatever knows which books have been set aside, yet the clairvoyant is reported as giving the gist of the passage she has selected sufficiently often to make the hypothesis of chance unplausible. In yet another kind of experiment the medium is handed some object whose history is unknown to all present ; it is alleged that sometimes detailed accounts of episodes in which it has been concerned are given. To explain these phenomena by the hypothesis of telepathy would plainly involve something like a central pool wherein the knowledge of all men is stored, a pool whence the medium is able to draw her knowledge. But this is so desperate a conjecture that very much more stringent conditions would be required to establish such occurrences as facts than are required for more ordinary cases of telepathy.

Dissociation. In some cases the mediumistic trance is a state of what is known as *dissociation*. The medium claims ordinarily to be ' controlled ' by an independent personality. It often appears to be that of a child. Now mild degrees of dissociation are not uncommon. Just as we can digest and at the same time learn to ride a bicycle, so when we have learned to ride we can continue on our way while arguing about birth-control. There is nothing pathological about this, but when the two streams of activity are such that one would normally inhibit the other, and the two cannot be combined into a coherent personality, an abnormal condition may arise. There is a surprisingly large number of people who, if they hold a pencil comfortably in their hand over a piece of paper, while reading a book or talking to others, find that after a little practice the pencil begins to move and write down more or less coherent script. This is known as automatic writing. A set of interests which has been repressed by normal consciousness is taking advantage of this channel of expression. In extreme cases this dissociated set of interests is complete enough to make up a minor personality, and it may be added that provision of the means of expression often favours the development of the disease.

Facial Asymmetry. Many people who have never heard of ' dissociation ' are aware that the faces of their friends are not the same on the right side as on the left ; and discussion frequently arises as to which side will come out best in a photograph. In extreme cases the disparity of expression is very marked, and insanity is often indicated by a cocking of one eyebrow. In normal people both halves of the forehead muscle work together, but in states of dissociation one half will work independently. Normally, too, the eyes are directed largely by impulses from the cortex of the opposite side, after the manner of a pair of horses' heads controlled as depicted in Fig. VIII ; but squint may indicate dissociation of this curious faculty of conjugate direction, and the imbalance involved may explain the distrust of many for people who squint as unreliable. Phrases such as 'double-faced', 'smiling on one

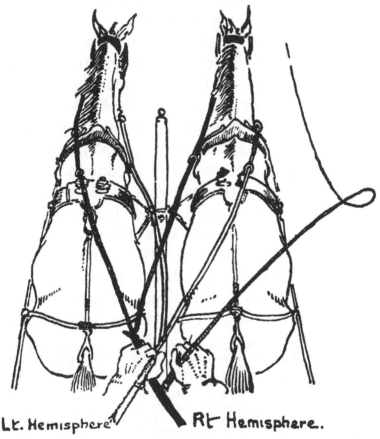

Lt. Hemisphere Rt Hemisphere.

FIG. VIII.

side of the face', or 'laughing on the wrong side', show a further recognition of this lack of co-ordination. The correlation of

R

squint with left-handedness, and the possibility of their origin in some infantile reaction to thwarting by a heavy father are now receiving attention from oculists who are conversant with psychology.

But the psychological bearing of asymmetry extends to the whole personality. In civilized man the *left* side of the brain (connected with the right side of the face and body) is usually the dominant hemisphere. Intellectual development (in right-handed people) depends on the potentialities and predominance of the left brain. The palmists express this by saying that the right hand (governed by the left brain) reveals what the owner has accomplished, while the left hand (governed by the right brain) shows his congenital equipment and inheritance.[1] Hence when a man rises by his own efforts we may expect

---

[1] A discussion of this distinction from a practical standpoint will be found in *The Hand and the Mind* (1928), by Mrs M. N. Laffan, chapter ii., and in due course physiologists may be able to throw light on other generalizations concerning the hand which palmists claim to have established.. The psychology of handwriting also raises many curious problems, such as those dealt with by Dr Macdonald Critchley in his *Mirror Writing* (1928). Not only are there persons who habitually write backwards with the left hand, like Leonardo da Vinci, but some, on occasion, even speak backwards ; and anyone in search of new psychological experiences cannot do better than experiment with the reversed gramophone first demonstrated by Sir Richard Paget, in December, 1928, at the Royal Institution, when Sir J. Forbes Robertson's rendering of " Hamlet's advice to the players " was re-rendered by the present writer in phonetic reverse.

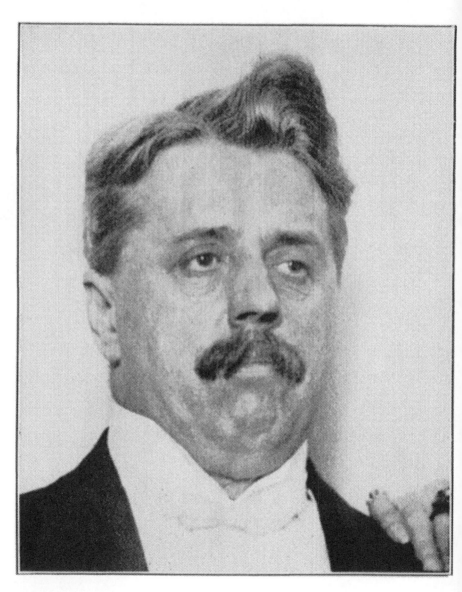

PLATE IV

to see his origins revealed in the left side of his face, his accomplishments in his right.

When two or more such personalities are unified (unilateral control) at a high level of development, we get the various forms of 'genius' which are associated with versatility and synthetic achievement. Thus in the portrait of the distinguished writer on the opposite page—who was also a discriminating and sagacious psychologist, though he found it more profitable to call his work fiction—the reader may imagine on the right hand side of the dotted line (the left side of the face) the penetrating humorist who created *The Card,* and on the other side the reflective artist whose *Old Wives' Tale* remains a landmark in literature. Facial asymmetry of this type is usually combined with pronounced right or left-handedness and those in whom it is most marked are often regarded by their less wayward friends as unaccountable and disturbing—" you never know where you are with them ". A different type of genius is found, though very rarely, in unified personalities with complete facial symmetry, both cerebral hemispheres being abnormally developed at a very high level: as for example in the well-known Stratford bust of

Shakespeare. Perfect symmetry of face on a low level (the left side of the brain having failed to develop above the right) is seen in certain idiots and criminals.

Alternating Personalities. A very striking form of dissociation may occur when the lack of co-ordination between two or more mental systems (whether from + Left or — Right or some more complicated disorder) is so great as to result in what is known as alternating or dual personality ; those fugues, or flights from reality, which occur in cases of hysteria. Certain drugs, notably alcohol and hashish, or the deep-breathing practices of the Yoga system, are artificial means of inducing them. A great part of the technique of the religions of antiquity was devoted to bringing about similar states, and to-day the trance medium is in many respects the lineal descendant of the Priestess of Apollo. In the trance the medium often utters strange cries, writhes and gesticulates. Raps and voices are heard in all parts of the room, and, strangest of all, physical objects are sometimes reported as moving, even with violence, beyond the medium's reach. Endeavours are, of course, made to control the movements of the medium's limbs, but the darkness or low illumination, and the hubbub that is usually declared to be essential, make any scientific judgment difficult. All that can be stated is that if such phenomena are genuine, physics, physiology, and psychology alike are very far from being able to explain them at present ; whether their verification would invalidate any particular view of the nature of the mind cannot, therefore, be decided. In any case such *séances* provide a valuable field for a study of the psychology of belief and testimony.[1]

Calculating Boys. The unconscious is often regarded as a source of all that is most marvellous in the mind. Certainly some of the performances of the very backward nine-year-old child Zerah Colburn, who could instantly declare the factors of six figure numbers and extract cube roots without a moment's hesitation, though entirely ignorant of the commonest rules of arithmetic, require a special explanation. When later on he discovered in part how the feat had been performed, the odd consequence was that he lost the capacity. Apparently at the age of

[1] One of the few scientific accounts of modern *séances*, in which the alleged production of ' ectoplasm ' is often a feature, will be found in *Psyche*, April, 1927 (vol. vii, No. 4)—constituting an exposure of the famous trance medium Willi Schneider.

six he had indulged in an enormous number of multiplication sums involving two figures, classifying the products by the last two digits. He then unconsciously remembered what numbers when multiplied together could yield products so ending. The power of finding factors and extracting roots seems to have depended upon this prodigious unconscious classification. G. P. Bidder, a calculator even more remarkable than Colburn, used similar methods, believed in multiplying from the left-hand corner, and never lost his capacity for lightning calculation in all forms. Two days before his death at the age of seventy-two the query was suggested : Taking the velocity of light at 190,000 miles per second, and the wave length of the red rays at 36,918 to an inch, how many of its waves must strike the eye in one second ? His friend, producing a pencil, was about to calculate the result, when Mr Bidder said : " You need not work it : the number of vibrations will be four hundred and forty-four billions, four hundred and thirty-three thousand six hundred and fifty-one millions, two hundred thousand ". This number written in figures is 444,433,651,200,000.[1]

[1] Hankin, *Common Sense and How to Acquire It*, 1925, p. 55.

A different kind of calculator was Jedediah Buxton, whose memory for figures was amazing, though he never learned more than the simple multiplication table. Though he was very slow and did little else in his whole life but multiplication, he failed to discover that the simplest way to multiply a number by 100 is to add oo. He talked freely whilst solving his problems, and could complete an unfinished problem three months later, taking it up where he left it. He remembered all the free drinks of beer he had had since he was twelve years of age; amounting to 5,116 pints received from 60 persons.

Musical Prodigies. Another precocious capacity which has naturally attracted attention is musical genius. Most of the great composers were remarkable for their early musical development, and in many cases exhibited astonishing gifts of discrimination and analysis. In his elaborate study of the powers of Erwin Nyiregyházi, to which we referred in Chapter IX, Dr Révész describes his analyses of the three chords

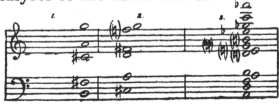

the first time they were played to him at
the age of seven.

The Inheritance of Genius. It is natural
to inquire how far special capacities are due
to inheritance and how far to early environment. But the usual antithesis between
heredity and environment is no longer justified. Modern genetics has shown that if
we could give the same education for many
generations to a number of different human
families, we should find that the characteristics resulting from education are inherited
characteristics in the same sense as are colour
of eyes and form of head. " Every creature, "
adds Professor H. S. Jennings, " has many
inheritances ; which one shall be realized
depending on the conditions under which it
develops ; but man is the creature that has
the greatest number of possible heritages.
Or, more accurately, men and other organisms
do not inherit their characteristics at all.
What their parents leave them are certain
packets of chemicals which under one set of
conditions produce one set of characters,
under other conditions produce other sets".

The Great Abnormals. It is useful to
realize how many of the greatest figures in
history have suffered from grave disabilities

and apparently congenital defects which might have been expected to debar them from worldly success. If St Paul suffered from contagious ophthalmia, as the late Dean Farrar held ; if Napoleon was a victim of Fröhlich's dystrophia adiposo-genitalis, as the late Dr Leonard Guthrie conclusively proved ; if Coleridge was an opium-addict, Dostoevski an epileptic, Nietzsche a martyr to migraine, and Darwin for thirty-six years lived a valetudinarian life (during which he published twenty-three volumes and fifty-one important scientific papers)—we should hesitate to regard good health and perfect normality as the first of human needs.

CHAPTER XVII

LOOKING FORWARD

THERE is no department of human activity in which psychology may not be of assistance or does not promise help. On the other hand, we must not in practical life, too often expect from psychology light upon topics which common sense cannot at least faintly illumine. Rather shall we find, reinforced and supported on a systematic basis, the fragmentary conclusions which shrewd and observant people have already reached.

Man's Protracted Infancy. We have seen in Chapter VIII that man, of all animals, has the longest period of infancy. He is the most incompetent in his early months, and has the most complex social environment to which to adapt himself. This is partly due to the immense extent of the social heritage carried by language and institutions, which is now quite beyond the attainment of the individual child without the aid of education. The whole effect of recent psychological discovery has been to confirm the view that the first three years of childhood are of overwhelming importance for the rest of life. The fixity of early trends, and the acquisition of modes of dealing with the environment which are transferred and reapplied to an ever wider circle of situations, make it clear that education too often begins only when one of its main tasks has been clumsily finished.

Doubtless there is a sense in which the child's first and best educator would be the ideal mother : but the records of child life in the past, in spite of notable exceptions, do not encourage us to envy those of our predecessors who survived the cradle ; and modern economic tendencies are making it more and more necessary to replace the guttering light of nature by a galaxy of well-considered principles and trained assistants. No one readily trusts himself in a car driven by an amateur for the first time. Yet we cheerfully leave a much more difficult undertaking in the hands of an unaided novice. If the modern mother has to be taught to keep the child's bottle clean, how much more does she need help in learning not to poison its mind with all those unnecessary fears and desires which are occupying the attention of psychiatrists to-day (Cf. Chapters X and XV).

School Education. Further, the study of suggestion shows that everyone with whom a child comes in contact is in these early years, as to a lesser extent throughout his life, an educator. Suggestion leads characteristically to imitation in the simplest sense. Barking dogs or whistling winds are imitated almost automatically. But later, so early as the second year, this imitation becomes a deliberate activity controlled by a desire to copy what other people are doing and guided by an explicit idea of what this is. The prodigious exercise in imitation, and the prestige which successful imitation thereby gains, are best seen in the acquisition of language. The slightest deviation from the linguistic conventions of the home circle is at once stamped out with a ruthlessness which only a student of phonetics, of dialects and comparative linguistic, can realize. The plasticity of the child's vocal habits and its zeal in imitation make this the golden moment for an initial training in the sounds of foreign languages. A similar linguistic opportunity occurs during adolescence, when those strange aberrations of interest in language for its own sake, the counterpart of the universal primitive belief in Word-magic, hold sway. The power of concentration on what may afterwards be regarded as dreary details is at its height between the ages of seven and seventeen, but at present, as a rule, little advantage is taken of these capacities otherwise than in the interests of formal training.

The Transfer of Training. The great problem thus arises, do formal exercises, whether in Latin Grammar, in Arithmetic, in Music, or in History, lead to mental development which can be transferred to other subject-matter? The present conclusion, based on methods of mental measurement to which we shall return, is on the whole negative. But of course everything turns upon the precise way in which the formal training is given. A blind fumbling without any goal in sight, animated by a vague hope of satisfying a largely incomprehensible demand, can teach nothing; and to-day unfortunately most people have cause to resent the loss of a valuable decade largely spent in such pursuits. A suitable epitaph

for many a teacher of the old school would
be :

> " Here lies One
> Who wasted All his Own time
> And Much of Other people's."

The Case Against Education. It is
hardly surprising, in view of the failure of
most schools to profit by the findings both
of common sense and psychology, that the
question, " Is school education doing more
harm than good ? " is still periodically raised
by headmasters of securely endowed institutions, as well as by employers and trade
unionists. There is, however, also the
consideration that in some way human beings
have to be inured to drudgery and unnecessary
toil, and that in this respect current education admirably fits a man for the world as
he will find it. But this is not an argument
of which educationists are proud ; and we
hear on all sides of the difficulty of finding
men and women able to take responsibility,
or to do anything they have not already
been repeatedly shown how to do.

Vocational Training. The cure for this,
from the point of view of the psychologist,
is either a formal education both wide enough
and conducted with sufficient insight (which

involves thinkers as teachers, small classes and a consequent tenfold increase in educational expenditure), or an adequate and enlightened scheme of vocational training. Any discussion of this choice, however, involves social and economic considerations which are outside the scope of the present work. Are we moving towards a general sharing out of unavoidable labour, or towards scientific discoveries and technical applications which will make highly trained intelligence the first essential?

Incentives. In any case the problem of incentives in education remains, and here the arguments presented by advocates of the vocational school are valid.[1] Without some concrete practical problem which is in itself arousing interest, the teacher must rely upon his own personality, upon comparatively feeble indirect inducements, or upon the competitive spirit. All these are motives which in comparison with a genuine interest in the work itself are of low educational value. The most reliable incentive, and the one most worth developing, is the pupil's own sense of his growing command of the subject; for this springs from the

---

[1] Kerschensteiner,. *The Schools and the Nation*, chap. vi.

self-regarding sentiment which is the nucleus of the personality. Thus a practical recommendation of some importance is that children should be encouraged constantly to measure their capacities not against those of others, but against their own at an earlier stage ; and in particular to reflect upon the means by which the improvement has been brought about. The reasonable confidence which this engenders is not to be confused with vanity, and is in fact the surest safeguard against it.

Mental Types. One of the points in psychology which is of most interest to the teacher concerns the recent work on types. The classifications of the past have dealt chiefly with intellectual differences, with contrasting attitudes to special kinds of objects. Thus we get Synthetic and Analytic minds, Intuitive and Logical, Romantic and Classic, Visual and Auditive, and so forth. Recently the speculations of Jung have received much attention. His classification forms a kind of chessboard with four horizontal divisions —sensation, intuition, feeling, and thinking —and two vertical divisions—extravert and introvert. Sensation and intuition are lower level forms of what at a higher stage of development appear as feeling and thinking. In this way eight main types are obtained. But since all these terms are used in special senses, and the whole classification is based on a theory of the collective unconscious and of primordial symbols, which have all the air of being emotive rather than precise forms of speech, the practical value of these types is problematic. Moreover, most people in the course of a day will find themselves fitting into several. Those who employ the terms ' extraverted ' and ' introverted ' in a broad sense as equivalent to ' practical ' and ' reflective ' might find the latter, and the many similar pairs which are already in current use, more profitable.

The ancient classification into the sanguine, melancholy, choleric, and phlegmatic suggests a more useful line of approach. Recent work on the internal secretions or hormones, though still in its initial stages, makes it probable that not only physique, but character also, is closely dependent on what is known as the endocrine balance. We dealt in Chapter XIV with one of the internal secretions, the adrenalin produced by the adrenal glands, but it should be noted that there are many other glands, of which the thyroid, the

S

pituitary, the thymus and the reproductive glands are the most important. The substances which they produce are carried in the blood-stream and vitally affect the growth and functioning of the tissues. Certain emotions such as fear, rage, and pain are known to be directly related to the discharge of adrenalin, and it seems likely that correlations may in due course be established for other secretions. Another hopeful line is that which relates certain types of physique with particular temperaments and capacities :

> " Let me have men about me that are fat ;
> Sleek-headed men, and such as sleep o' nights :
> Yon Cassius has a lean and hungry look ;
> He thinks too much : such men are dangerous."

Cassius, in the language of Kretschmer [1] who is chiefly responsible for the alarming vocabulary of this subject, was a ' schizothyme '. Cæsar would have desired him to be more of a ' cyclothyme ' !

Moreover, every classification of types must take note of racial and national differences. This is not the place to raise the fascinating topic of man's animal ancestry and the

---

[1] *Physique and Character*, 1925, p. 208. A valuable discussion of these distinctions will be found in E. Miller's *Types of Mind and Body* (1926) ; while the possible effect of the conditions under which man obtained his food during the first million years of pre-history is suggestively considered in R. Lowe Thompson's *The Hunter in our Midst* (1926).

traces of pre-anthropoid evolution in the human organism as a possible basis for the differentiation of types ; but it may be noted that recent work on racial origins has made it probable that the three chief stems of humanity, the White, the Black, and the Yellow (Shem, Ham, and Japheth), are allied, respectively, to the Chimpanzee, the Gorilla, and the Orang [1] ; and further, that they are far more intermingled than we suppose.

Mental Tests. It is these multiple possibilities of type differences in one apparently pure stock which make such wholesale methods as are used in mental tests of less practical use than is often supposed. The devoted labours of the vast army of mental testers are slowly laying the foundations for an objective method of comparison, of which the ultimate scientific advantages may be great. It is useful to have a standard even if we do not know what it is a standard of ; since it is always possible that this may be discovered. But meanwhile the use of crude ' efficiency ' methods in place of the more traditional and leisurely ways of judging ability and desirability is suitable rather for economic and military crises than for a

[1] Crookshank, *The Mongol in our Midst* (2nd edition, 1925).

civilization which prides itself upon its complexity and its refinement. There is much to be said for the quick lunch ; but there are those who prefer to treat themselves more sympathetically. In particular, such methods are apt to be unjust to the very individuals on whom the future may most depend. Even as things are the genius is too often regarded as an imbecile ; mental tests in many cases *prove* him to be one. But what can be tested is unfortunately not always what is most valuable. Few experimenters would deny this, but the temptation to make practical social applications in conformity with current standards is strong.

The Future of Communication. The reader will have noticed the stress laid upon language in these pages. The centre of interest in psychology has of recent years shifted considerably, and the symbolizing activities of the mind are more and more becoming its main concern. In some quarters there is actually a tendency to overestimate the importance of the language factor. Many who regard thinking as silent talking overlook the fact that one of the chief practical problems of psychology is to distinguish verbal from non-verbal thinkers—another, perhaps fundamental, division of the types which are discussed above. And even among verbalizers we must distinguish those who are at the mercy of their expressions from those who are not, a distinction of great practical importance in all discussion. There are some people, and those not the least eminent, who can only be persuaded to change their opinion when they are presented with a formal rearrangement of their own vocabulary, while others can grasp a point, however it is put. In university and adult education generally this is of supreme importance, and the technique by which men can be delivered from the bondage of set phrases in earlier years is slowly being evolved. One of the first tasks of those who appreciate the bearing of this aspect of the psychology of thinking on human progress must be to make conscious the manifold strivings towards such a technique, which are found, for example, in grammatical reform movements, in the study of semantics, in new methods of language teaching, and even in simplified spelling. ' Orthology ' is a convenient term by means of which these various converging tendencies may be focussed.

Another sign of this endeavour is seen in

the steady decline in psychology of the traditional type of argumentation in which the disputants revolve patiently each in his own closed system of linked definitions, and keep in touch with one another only through the fact that each is using the same word, though in different senses. The freedom with which psycho-analysts, behaviorists, and even traditionalists are busy coining new vocabularies is on the whole an encouraging symptom, since it at least prevents the general student who is linguistically plastic from becoming prematurely encaged in too narrow a symbolic system.

But if this happy result is to ensue it is essential that men become word-conscious. A similar multiplication of technicalities is occurring in all the sciences, and is particularly embarrassing in the social sciences. It may lead to great difficulties if not to general unintelligibility and a sterilizing isolation of specialists, unless psychology comes to the rescue by inducing a new attitude towards speech based on an understanding of what is happening when we speak. The important point is to remember that what any thought is ' of ' or ' about ' (its Referent, to use a convenient technicality) and the formulation of the thought, must never be confused. Every statement is translatable, and translation should form a chief part of intellectual training at all stages ; not only translation from foreign languages into our own, though this is at present probably the most valuable part of the general curriculum, but also, and still more urgently, translation from one formulation to another within the bounds of our native tongue. By this means we may best become word-conscious, that is, become able to look beyond our forms of speech to the things we are talking about. A truly sagacious Dictator would make it his first business to create a Word-conscious Proletariat.

The Need for Conscious Control. This need for increased conscious control of the machinery of life is even more evident when we turn to the influence which modern psychology is exerting in medicine. Why have we this sudden universal emphasis on the psychological origin of so much mental and physical disease ? Is it not because the problems of existence which a little while ago were so simply solved, have, with the increasing complexity of modern civilization, begun to put a strain upon the old mechanisms ?

Just as we should take over conscious control of the Words which have set men chasing after so many unrealities, in the same way we must learn to take charge of our Minds. We are beginning to realize, with the aid of the doctor, that our neuralgia, our headache, our migraine, our dyspepsia, and even our phthisis, are, no less than the phobias, the hysterias, the anxieties, and the other neuroses which loom so large in the contemporary social picture, as often as not ways in which we are dodging some awkward situation or decision. We have been evading the issue. We have lost touch with reality. And again, just as we evade the personal problem, so civilization as a whole is evading the cosmic issue. Vaguely apprehensive that the old solutions in their traditional form can no longer be squared with the facts, we either look wistfully backwards, or compromise with some morbific phantom which we conjure up to screen us from the abyss. But we must dare to be wise, and the way to wisdom lies through knowledge of ourselves. The facts which we can least afford to neglect are those which it is the object of psychology to present.

BIBLIOGRAPHY

The following books have been selected as representative of modern psychological opinion in the various fields covered in outline by the present work, and as likely to be of service to the general reader for the further study of contemporary psychology.

Adler, Alfred, *Individual Psychology.*
Baudouin, *Suggestion and Autosuggestion.*
Bayliss, *Principles of General Physiology.*
Bechterev, *General Principles of Human Reflexology.*
Bergson, *Matter and Memory.*
Bernal, *The World, the Flesh, and the Devil.*
Bernfeld, *Psychology of the Infant.*
Boring, *History of Experimental Psychology.*
Brett, *History of Psychology* (3 vols).
Broad, *Mind and Its Place in Nature.*
Burt, *The Young Delinquent.*
Cannon, *Bodily Changes in Pain, Hunger, Fear and Rage.*
Chadwick, *Difficulties in Child Development.*
Child, *Physiological Foundations of Behavior.*
Collins, *Colour Blindness.*
Crookshank, *Migraine and other Common Neuroses.*
        The Mongol in our Midst.
De Sanctis, *Religious Conversion.*
Dewey, *Human Nature and Conduct.*
Ellis, *The World of Dreams.*
        Psychology of Sex (6 vols).
Fox, *Educational Psychology.*
Flugel, *A Hundred Years of Psychology.*
Freud, *Collected Papers* (4 vols).
        A General Introduction to Psychoanalysis.
        The Interpretation of Dreams.

Gillespie, *Hypochondria.*
Gordon, *Personality.*
Gregory, *The Nature of Laughter.*
Hamilton, *The Art of Interrogation.*
Hart, *The Psychology of Insanity.*
Hatfield, *The Conquest of Thought by Invention.*
Helmholtz, *Sensations of Tone.*
Herrick, *Neurological Foundations of Animal Behavior.*
Hobhouse, *Mind in Evolution.*
Jaensch, *Eidetic Imagery.*
James, *Principles of Psychology.*
Jung, *Psychological Types.*
Kellogg, *The Ape and the Child.*
Koffka, *The Growth of the Mind.*
Köhler, *The Mentality of Apes.*
Kretschmer, *Physique and Character.*
Ladd-Franklin, *Colour and Colour Theories.*
Lange, *The History of Materialism.*
Lashley, *Brain Mechanisms and Intelligence.*
Leuba, *The Psychology of Religious Mysticism.*
McCurdy, *The Psychology of Emotion.*
McDougall, *Outline of Psychology.*
           Physiological Psychology.
Miller (N.), *The Child in Primitive Society.*
Mitchell, *Structure and Growth of the Mind.*
Morgan, *Instinct and Experience.*
Murphy, *An Historical Introduction to Modern Psychology.*
Ogden (C. K.) and Richards, *The Meaning of Meaning.*
Ogden (Robert M.), *Hearing.*
O'Shea, *Mental Development and Education.*
Parsons, *Colour Vision.*
Pavlov, *Conditional Reflexes.*
Perrier, *The Earth before History.*
Piéron, *Thought and the Brain.*
           Principles of Experimental Psychology.

Pole, *The Philosophy of Music.*
Pratt, *The Religious Consciousness.*
Prince, *The Dissociation of a Personality.*
Révész, *The Psychology of a Musical Prodigy.*
Richards, *Principles of Literary Criticism.*
     Practical Criticism.
Rignano, *The Psychology of Reasoning.*
Rivers, *Conflict and Dream.*
Russell, *The Analysis of Mind.*
Semon, *Mneme.*
Shand, *The Foundations of Character.*
Sherrington, *The Integrative Action of the Nervous System.*
Stefansson, *The Standardization of Error.*
Stern, G., *Meaning and Change of Meaning.*
Stern, W. *The Psychology of Early Childhood.*
Stout, *Analytic Psychology* (2 vols).
Thomson, *Instinct, Intelligence and Character.*
Thorndike, *The Psychology of Learning.*
Tischner, *Telepathy and Clairvoyance.*
Troland, *The Mystery of Mind.*
Trotter, *The Instincts of the Herd.*
Van der Hoop, *Character and the Unconscious.*
Warden, *Outline of Comparative Psychology.*
Watson, *Behaviorism.*
Weiss, *A Theoretical Basis of Human Behavior.*
Wilson, *Aphasia.*
Woodworth, *Psychology.*

INDEX